Men's Health

Life Improvement Guides®

Guy Knowledge

Skills, Tricks, and
Techniques That
Your Father Meant
to Teach You—
But Probably Didn't

by Larry Keller, Christian Millman,
and the Editors of Men's Health Books

Rodale Press, Inc.
Emmaus, Pennsylvania

Copyright © 1999 by Rodale Press, Inc.

Illustrations copyright © 1999 by Alan Baseden, John Kocon, and Bryon Thompson

"The Last Laugh" on page 103 was adapted and reprinted from *The Book of Lists* by David Wallechinsky and Amy Wallace. Copyright © 1993 by David Wallechinsky and Amy Wallace. Reprinted by permission of Ed Victor Ltd.

"Catchin' Out for Freedom" by Guitar Whitey on page 108 was adapted from *Around the Jungle Fire*. Copyright © 1994 by Cliff Williams. Reprinted by permission of The Hobo Press.

Other titles in the *Men's Health Life Improvement Guides* series:

Command Respect	*Food Smart*	*Maximum Style*	*Sex Secrets*	*Symptom Solver*
Death Defiers	*Good Loving*	*Money Savvy*	*Stress Blasters*	*Vitamin Vitality*
Fight Fat	*Healing Power*	*Powerfully Fit*	*Stronger Faster*	

Library of Congress Cataloging-in-Publication Data

Keller, Larry.
   Guy knowledge : skills, tricks, and techniques that your father
meant to teach you—but probably didn't / by Larry Keller, Christian
Millman, and the editors of Men's Health books.
      p.   cm. — (Men's health life improvement guides)
   Includes index.
   ISBN 0–87596–507–5 paperback
   1. Men—Attitudes. 2. Men—Conduct of life. 3. Identity
(Psychology) 4. Men—Psychology. I. Millman, Christian.
II. Men's health (Magazine) III. Title. IV. Series.
HQ1090.K46 1999
305.31—dc21   99–18115

Distributed to the book trade by St. Martin's Press

2 4 6 8 10 9 7 5 3 1   paperback

Visit us on the Web at www.menshealthbooks.com or call us toll-free at (800) 848-4735

OUR PURPOSE

*"We inspire and enable people to improve
their lives and the world around them."*

Guy Knowledge Editorial Staff

Managing Editor: **Jack Croft**

Writers: **Larry Keller, Christian Millman**

Contributing Writers: **Stephen C. George, Jan Eickmeier, Mary Kittel, Deanna Moyer, Deborah Pedron**

Associate Art Director: **Charles Beasley**

Cover Designer and Series Art Director: **Tanja Lipinski-Cole**

Series Designer: **John Herr**

Cover Photographer: **Mitch Mandel**

Part Opener Illustrator: **Bryon Thompson**

Chapter Opener Illustrator: **Alan Baseden**

Technical Illustrator: **John Kocon Illustration**

Associate Research Manager: **Jane Unger Hahn**

Lead Researcher: **Deanna Moyer**

Editorial Researchers: **Lori Davis, Mary Kittel, Mary S. Mesaros, Kathryn Piff, Elizabeth Price, Staci Sander**

Senior Copy Editor: **Amy K. Kovalski**

Layout Designer: **Donna G. Rossi**

Associate Studio Manager: **Thomas P. Aczel**

Manufacturing Coordinators: **Brenda Miller, Jodi Schaffer, Patrick T. Smith**

Rodale Active Living Books

Vice President and Publisher: **Neil Wertheimer**

Editorial Director: **Michael Ward**

Writing Director: **Brian Paul Kaufman**

Marketing Director: **Janine Slaughter**

Product Marketing Manager: **Kris Siessmayer**

Book Manufacturing Director: **Helen Clogston**

Manufacturing Managers: **Eileen F. Bauder, Mark Krahforst**

Research Manager: **Ann Gossy Yermish**

Copy Manager: **Lisa D. Andruscavage**

Production Manager: **Robert V. Anderson Jr.**

Office Manager: **Roberta Mulliner**

Office Staff: **Jacqueline Dornblaser, Julie Kehs, Suzanne Lynch, Mary Lou Stephen**

Photo Credits

Page 152: **Courtesy of Maggie Smith**

Page 154: **Corbis**

Page 156: **Courtesy of KingWorld**

Page 158: **Courtesy of Richard Radstone/MGM**

Page 160: **Ron Posey/Courtesy of Clive Cussler**

Back flap: **Alinari/Art Resource, NY**

Contents

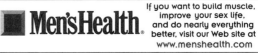

Introduction

Knowledge Is Good

He was rich and powerful. The founder of his own town. The father of the modern American lead pencil. For most men, that would have been enough. But not for Emil Faber. Despite all of his success, the one thing that gnawed at the fictional business titan was that he never graduated from college. So in 1904, he founded Faber College. Years later, this venerable institution of higher learning would be immortalized in that classic of cinema verité, *National Lampoon's Animal House*.

In the film's opening scene, the camera slowly zooms in on the statue of Faber that graces the campus. Inscribed on the statue are the words that have inspired generations of students and filmgoers: "Knowledge is good."

Yes, it is. Pointy-headed intellectuals may snicker at Faber's homespun wisdom, but let me tell you, those three simple words convey a profound truth: Knowing stuff is better than not knowing stuff. Especially for guys.

That's why we wrote *Guy Knowledge*. Because let's face it: With the notable exceptions of learning how to crush a beer can on your forehead or convert a wrecked Lincoln into a Deathmobile to ruin the homecoming parade, college is the last place you'll find the kind of knowledge that men really crave.

So what, precisely, is guy knowledge? It's knowing how to do the things that men are *expected* to know how to do. Like changing the car's oil. Or fixing a leaky faucet. Or getting rid of spiders, mice, and other pests. They don't teach you this stuff in college, and it doesn't get passed along genetically with the Y chromosome. Yet, despite lip service from the politically correct, gender-neutral crowd, when some furry little rodent scurries across the floor, it's automatically the man's job to get rid of it.

Guy knowledge is also knowing how to do the things that men actually *want* to know how to do. Like mixing drinks with a bartender's flair and giving a toast that leaves guests alternately laughing and weeping. Like blowing a fastball by someone the way Nolan Ryan did. Like not only getting on the air on talk radio but also having something smart to say when you do. And that's just at play. At work, guys want to know how to get a raise, a promotion, or a leave of absence. Maybe even all three, preferably at the same time.

It's all here, in this handy, entertaining guide. You'll learn how to be a man's man—not to mention a ladies' man. Some of this stuff is practical, and some of it is admittedly whimsical. Okay, so the odds of quitting your day job and running off to join the circus—or, better yet, running off to exotic locales to snap pictures of gorgeous models in skimpy bikinis—are pretty damn slim. Still, it would be nice to know how you *could* do it. And maybe you'll never be able to tip with the panache of Sinatra, throw a spiral with the finesse of Elway, or play poker with the nerve of Cool Hand Luke. But armed with *Guy Knowledge*, you'll be able to do those things—and much more—better than you can today. And that's a start.

We subtitled this book *Skills, Tricks, and Techniques That Your Father Meant to Teach You—But Probably Didn't*. That's not a knock on your old man. After all, he was a guy, too—scrambling to make a living, raise a family, and maybe have a little fun. When you get right down to it, that's the main thing that *Guy Knowledge* will do for you—make your life a little more fun.

It may have been a laugh line in *Animal House*, but it turns out that Emil Faber was right: Knowledge *is* good. And this book is rich with it.

Jack Croft

Jack Croft
Managing Editor, *Men's Health* Books

Part One

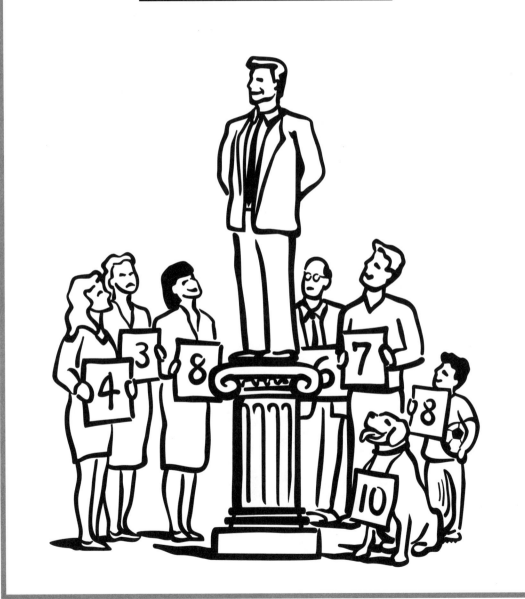

What Men Know

How to Be a Stone Age Man in a Space Age World

Scientists have now confirmed what we have long suspected: We are cavemen living in a modern world. And Adrian Targett is the living proof.

DNA tests conducted by Oxford University scientists in the spring of 1997 found that Targett, a history teacher, is a direct descendant of Cheddar Man, a 9,000-year-old skeleton found less than a mile from Targett's home in England.

"My wife says that's why I like my steak rare," quips Targett.

But Targett—and the rest of us red-blooded males, for that matter—has far more in common with his fossilized forefather than a taste for red meat.

"It's very difficult to find differences between someone who lived 10,000 years ago and someone at present," explains David Glenn Smith, Ph.D., professor of anthropology at the University of California, Davis. Dr. Smith is an expert in a Cheddar Man peer—Kennewick Man, a 9,300-year-old skeleton found in the state of Washington.

"Emotionally and intellectually, we evolved to our present form a very long time ago," continues Dr. Smith.

But make no mistake, we proffer no apologies for our primitive wiring—we relish it. Manhood gives us ancient delights. We proudly bay at the moon. We drag our knuckles, leave our toenails untrimmed, and grunt

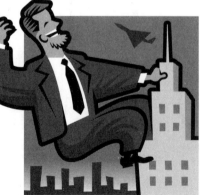

with glee. And, for years immemorial, we've taught our sons to do the same.

We are imprinted with Pleistocene memories, says Dr. Smith—memories left over from the birth of mankind that make us act and respond much as our primitive ancestors did.

But just as we hold the traits of a caveman, so did he have imbedded within him the genetic blueprint of a modern man. Ancient man held in him a noble, greater side, as do his sons of today. "Men strive," says George Hartlaub, M.D., associate clinical professor of psychiatry at the University of Colorado Health Sciences Center in Denver. "We always move, we always look for the better way. That is profound in us."

That drive has led men to scale Mount Everest simply because it's there, and to descend to the ocean's floor to find the Titanic. It has inspired and informed Shakespeare's sonnets, Emerson's mystical meditations, and Chandler's hard-boiled prose. It has given us the Sistine Chapel, the Taj Mahal, and the Empire State Building. It has blessed us with lasting images of Babe Ruth at bat, Joe Montana with the ball and less than two minutes on the clock, Michael Jordan soaring to heights that no one else could even imagine, and Muhammad Ali floating like a butterfly and stinging like a bee.

It is, in a very real sense, what makes us men.

Modern Times

As much as we enjoy our male heritage, this simple fact remains: Although we're virtually identical to our long-dead forefathers, the world around us bears little resemblance to theirs. We require an amazing number of skills to wend our way through modern life.

Famed science fiction writer Robert Heinlein put it this

way: "A human being should be able to change a diaper, plan an invasion, butcher a hog, conn a ship, design a building, write a sonnet, balance accounts, build a wall, set a bone, comfort the dying, take orders, give orders, cooperate, act alone, solve equations, analyze a new problem, pitch manure, program a computer, cook a tasty meal, fight efficiently, die gallantly. Specialization is for insects."

While there's not much call these days for planning an invasion (except for the occasional midnight raid on the refrigerator) or pitching manure (pitching woo, sure), you get the idea. No man is complete without a solid arsenal of guy skills to call his own.

Fortunately, most of these required skills can be lumped into several major categories.

Sex

We talk about it, think about it, dream about it. Sex speaks to the essence of manhood. It is the procreative urge, the siren song of nature, a most ancient want.

Here's what we know about sex.

- It's important to us. So essential is sex to our well-being that we often find ourselves cheerless in a relationship without it. "A couple with a good sex life finds that it accounts for about 10 percent of their happiness," says Fred E. Stickle, Ph.D., coordinator of counseling programs at Western Kentucky University in Bowling Green and a certified sex therapist. "But a couple with a bad sex life finds that it accounts for about 90 percent of their unhappiness."

- It's different for us. From the drop of the flag, a man can complete his sexual experience in about 2.8 minutes. "That doesn't mean they always do it, but that's the capability," says Dr.

> # This We Know
>
> **We hold these truths to be self-evident.**
>
> - **Just because we're adults now doesn't mean we can't actively seek out the banana with the sticker on it.**
> - **Our penises are *never* to be referred to as cute.**
> - **The fashion czars be damned—paisley ties will never go out of style for the simple reason that nothing else hides food stains as well.**
> - **A true barber never has the word *curls* in his shop's name.**
> - **Just because we know how to replace a belt in a washing machine doesn't mean we know how to load it.**
> - **There are two kinds of women—the kind you suck your gut in for and the kind you don't.**
> - **We're not being deliberately nasty when we leave the toilet seat up. If we were being deliberately nasty, we'd take it *off*.**
> - **Iced coffee makes about as much sense to us as hot peanut butter.**

Stickle. For a woman, the capability is 13.6 minutes. "It's virtually impossible to speed the woman up," he adds. So guess who needs to slow down?

- We dread being unable to do it. One survey found that middle-aged men would rather be deaf or blind than impotent. And when the impotence drug Viagra was introduced to American men, it spread like wildfire. Former U.S. Senator and presidential hopeful Bob Dole couldn't even wait until the official release—he was one of the men who took part in the trials.

- We want to be good at it. Despite the popular male-bashing stereotypes promulgated by TV sitcoms and women's magazines, most of us want to be good lovers. We want sex to be deeply satisfying and deliciously fun for our partners as well as ourselves.

Work

"Far and away the best prize that life offers is the chance to work hard at work worth doing," said President Theodore Roosevelt in a 1903 Labor Day speech.

This sentiment spans generations and even social philosophies. "Work is life, you know, and without it, there's nothing but fear and insecurity," said singer and 1960s icon John Lennon.

Here's what we know about work.

• It defines us. So important is our work, says Dr. Hartlaub, that we often base much of our identity on what we do for a living. Case in point: It's usually the first thing we inquire about when we meet another man—so, what do you do? We can even die without it. "A lot of men retire and there's nothing left," says Dr. Stickle.

• It's in our genes. "It's absolutely true that most men equate manhood with being a provider," says Dr. Hartlaub. You can't help it. It goes back to those Pleistocene memories we were talking about earlier. In psychiatry, it's called procedural memory—the hardwiring of our brains, our thoughts, the stuff that we don't even have words for.

• We bring it home. When there's grief in our jobs, there's almost always grief in our personal lives. "It's a big, big deal when guys lose their jobs or when there's work stress," says Dr. Hartlaub. Even in the days of dual-income households, we still can't stand to be unemployed.

• We like it. At least most of us do. Work is far from being all grim, serious stuff. The business magazine *Inc.* and the Gallup Organization found that 72 percent of Americans in the workforce were satisfied with their jobs.

Family

We tread a fine line here. A line that gets us in trouble with our significant others sometimes. Family is unquestionably vital to us. But sometimes we get so wrapped up in work that we forget the reason why we work so hard—to give our families the best things in life. We forget that the best thing, as far as they're concerned, is us, says Dr. Stickle.

Here's what we know about family.

• We're learning. More and more of us are coming to the conclusion that being involved in family life to a greater extent is really where it's at, says Dr. Stickle. "This doesn't mean that the career isn't important," he notes. "Just that we're realizing that it's helpful to hinge some of our self-esteem on a healthy family life."

• We need it. No one can call your bluff or see through your smoke screens like a member of your family. Brothers, sisters, fathers, mothers—they've known you longer than anyone. You may be a big shot at work, but you're a kid brother to someone who still likes to put you in a smelly-armpit headlock. We need that to keep us grounded and to put life in perspective.

• We're a necessary component. Study after study has shown the incredible benefits of a man being involved with his family. His kids do better all-around, his wife is happier and less likely to start dating Larry King. And he's happier. The days of dad and husband disappearing to his armchair, study, or neighborhood bar are fading. And no one is more pleased by the change than men.

Fun

"Men are but children of a larger growth," wrote the English poet John Dryden 300 years ago. This statement is equally applicable today, says Dr. Stickle. We still crave toys, gadgets, and gizmos. That adventurous spirit that caused us to cross vast oceans and dark expanses of space drives us to experience new things and see new sights. We love to laugh, and we wouldn't be able to communicate if jokes were suddenly outlawed.

Simply put, we want—no, we expect and demand—to have fun until the day we die. And the best part is that the more fun you have in life—the more active and involved you are—the longer it's likely to be until you cash in your chips at the big poker game in the sky.

Here's what we know about fun.

• It's a required activity. "Having a good sense of humor and the ability to have fun is a powerful tool in being successful in life," says Paul E. McGhee, Ph.D., a psychologist and president of the Laughter Remedy, a corporate consulting firm in Montclair, New Jersey, that offers programs on humor and laughter in the workplace.

• It's everywhere. Men incorporate fun into most things they do. Hence, pick-up sports, whoopie cushions, and even the fact that you take a different route to work to make it more interesting. Our love of fun colors our workday, strengthens our friendships, and even makes us better fathers.

The Tools to Do the Job

You wouldn't build a shed with a plastic hammer. You wouldn't hike the Appalachian trail in a pair of rubber boots. You wouldn't pursue the woman of your dreams with the social graces of a squid. Being a man requires premium, grade-A, top-notch tools.

That's what you hold in your hands. This guide represents the tools and skills you need to be a Stone Age man in a Space Age world. A man of style, ability, strength, common sense, and above all, good humor.

Read on, friend. Read on.

Love, Work, and Bras

Meet Jeffrey Bruce. For 10 years, he labored in a real estate job that he came to loathe. Now he has, arguably, the greatest job in the world. Based in Palo Alto, California, he's what is known as an underwear stylist. What that means is that he works with some of the world's most beautiful models and gets paid to wrangle their underwear into perfect position for photo shoots.

Now imagine making good money to smooth out the cleavage of and position stunningly attractive women. Toss on top of that the exotic locales around the world that Bruce gets sent to. He can be found plying his trade, clasps in hand, from the streets of Paris to the tropical beaches of the Pacific.

"I love doing it. It's novel. It's cool. It's unusual," he says. No kidding.

Making the jump from real estate to underwear took guts, admits Bruce, especially since there are only a handful of people who do what he does. "I took a risk and it paid off. It taught me an incredible lesson. Work goes beyond work," he says.

It's not all fun and flesh, though. Bruce does have a few pitfalls to contend with. For one thing, he carries a black bag with him on all his out-of-town calls. In it are stockings, tape, binder clips, bras, and a silky woman's robe. And something always sets off the alarm when he goes through airport security.

"At first, I was horrified," he admits. "They would start pulling things out. There's always a line behind me. People are staring." He used to try to offer an explanation.

"I don't even bother now."

What Other Men Expect You to Know

How to Be a Man's Man

We want to introduce you to a real man. His name is Wade L. Smith, and he's from Caldwell County in North Carolina.

On a horrifying day in 1998, Smith was standing in his bathroom, shaving, when a tornado touched down around his home. Through the window, he watched his 1,500-pound bull sliding across a field. Then the roof blew off.

Smith ran down into his basement with his dog. After the winds finished whipping his belongings into oblivion, Smith came out to survey the damage, his hair flecked with bits of pink insulation. What was his response as he looked at the remnants of his home and hearth?

"I didn't realize I had so much junk," said Smith.

"That's just an ideal response," explains Dr. Paul E. McGhee, president of the Laughter Remedy, a corporate consulting firm that offers programs on humor and laughter in the workplace. It's not that it belittles the gravity of the situation, says Dr. McGhee. It's that it typifies a response that virtually all men admire—coolness in the face of calamity, humor in the throes of tragedy, grace under fire.

Or, as Smith puts it, "When all you have left is your ring and your underwear, you'd better hold on to your sense of humor."

Think about the men you admire for a second. Think about what it is in them that you admire. Mentally make a list of some of the attributes they have.

Now, turn it around. Those things that you like so much are also the characteristics they expect from you.

The Right Stuff

According to a survey done by DYG, a group that tracks social trends, the following attributes are some of the things that men say they admire most in another man. They're listed in the order they were rated.

He's dependable. Perhaps the most important trait that one man looks for in another is this: If he tells you he's going to do something, he does it. Come hell or high water. Among men, there really is no higher compliment than "He's a man of his word."

"This is just a bedrock of the male code," says Ronald F. Levant, Ed.D., dean of the Center for Psychological Studies at Nova Southeastern University in Fort Lauderdale and coauthor of *Masculinity Reconstructed.*

He's honest. This is a direct corollary of being dependable: You know that you can trust a guy to give you a straight answer. "The need to trust is such a basic human emotion," says Dr. Levant.

He rolls up his sleeves and helps out. There's an addendum to this—he also doesn't brag about how hard he has worked. "I hear men who do one thing around the house and expect to be thanked up and down for it," says Western Kentucky University's Dr. Fred E. Stickle.

He has a good relationship with friends and family. Yes, we admire men who work hard. But we also know that there is more to life than work, and that family and friends make much of what we have to put up with worthwhile.

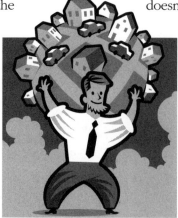

A man's man has found the correct balance of work, family, and friends, says Dr. Stickle. Who cares how good a guy you are if all anyone ever sees is your backside headed to work?

He has a sense of humor. Fortunately, this one often comes naturally to us. "When men get together, there's always a lot of laughter," says Dr. McGhee. Men enjoy wisecracking and joke telling. "We're also very good at poking fun at others," he says. But that's a two-way street that you better be able to navigate. "A lot of us are good at dishing it out but not very good at taking it," he continues. There's a term for that—poor sport. Don't be one.

He's authentic, not phony. We don't expect you to be perfect—far from it. Just don't pretend to be something you're not. "It's a high concern with men to not be bogus. We have to know that a guy means what he says and says what he means for him to win our trust," says the University of Colorado Health Sciences Center's Dr. George Hartlaub, who was a collaborator on the book *Men: A Translation for Women.*

He's a "regular guy." You hear this term all the time. But just what does it mean? Here's an example. "I created a revolving shooting target out of Barbra Streisand albums and a 12-volt motor," says Todd von Hoffman, coauthor of *The von Hoffman Brothers' Big Damn Book of Sheer Manliness.* "Barbra's great because all of her albums feature these huge head shots of her." It's even more fun, adds von Hoffman, when he attaches exploding caps to the back of the album, near her nose. "If you hit the nose, the whole thing goes sky high," he says. That's being a regular guy.

Those are the characteristics that other men rated most highly. The two characteristics

Reining In a Wayward Brother

Sometimes we go back on our word, sometimes we act like arrogant buffoons, sometimes we blame our teammates for fumbling the ball. If it becomes a habit, we go from acting like a jerk to being one. "We've all done it," explains the University of Colorado Health Sciences Center's Dr. George Hartlaub, who was a collaborator on the book *Men: A Translation for Women.*

As men, it's our responsibility to try to bring our errant brothers back into the fold before they become permanent outcasts, says Dr. Hartlaub. Plus, we hope they would do the same for us. So, how do we reach out to a fellow guy who stands outside the boundaries of the male code? Easy, the same way we wrestle—mano-a-mano.

"Men need a personal invitation from another man," Dr. Hartlaub says. "It's some kind of a man thing where we don't feel welcome unless we're approached personally."

So if you know someone who has strayed from the fold, invite him to a poker game or a ball game or out for a couple of beers. Then, call him on whatever jerklike behavior has made him an outcast. Directly and honestly. He may not listen, but at least he'll know that the guys are looking out for him, and that it's up to him whether he stays or goes.

that mattered the least to other guys may surprise you. They were making lots of money and being high-powered. That, says Dr. Levant, may be because men are highly competitive and it irks us to see men who are more successful than ourselves. Of course, it also could mean that we've seen enough first-class jerks making lots of money in high-powered jobs to know that those things don't make a man successful in the eyes of other men.

What Women Expect You to Know

How to Be a Ladies' Man

We've pondered this question in the driving rain, beating our palms against a locked door. We've furrowed our brows from deep within the doghouse. We've scratched our heads in confusion as the third day of sullen silence wears slowly on.

What, we ask the gods, the skies, the bottom of our beer glasses, do women expect from us, anyway? Fortunately, there is a very simple answer—one that many of us have overlooked.

"Too much," says the University of Colorado Health Sciences Center's Dr. George Hartlaub, who was a collaborator on the book *Men: A Translation for Women.* Perhaps we should be flattered, but the fact remains that women just give us too much credit. "They tend to look to us for more than we can offer, and they're almost uniformly disappointed in us," he says.

So what are we supposed to do about it? Compromise. You know what that is. You do it every time you eat at the employee cafeteria.

Blame this need to compromise on the changing world. In days gone by, every woman was part of a close-knit community of other women. Namely, her mother, her sisters, and all the old ladies in the village with great long whiskers on their chins. They worked side by side, chatted up a storm, and were happy. Now, the woman

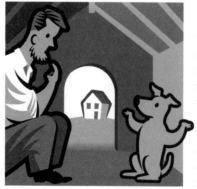

you're with probably lives far from her family, works full-time, and has traded in all those women for just you. So she's compromising big time, too.

"Women need to get a lot of what are called intimacy needs from other women," Dr. Hartlaub says. Hold on, put your camera away. He isn't talking about sex. He's talking about those intimate heart-to-hearts that she keeps coming after you for. With her support structure missing, she's looking to you to fill in. Too bad you're woefully unprepared.

The Toughest Questions on Earth

How many times have you been kicking back in your favorite BarcaLounger, enjoying the blissful silence, when the first dreaded question comes crashing down? "Honey, what are you thinking?" Women expect you to know how to answer this.

What to do, what to do? Do you make something up? To her, long periods of silence are a sign of important brooding. Do you let her in on the fact that you really weren't thinking anything and take the chance that she'll get mad because you never want to tell her what's on your mind?

"They don't get it," Dr. Hartlaub says. "Meanwhile, we're thinking about how come Elway didn't throw on third and long, or that we really have to get up and have a piss."

Compromise. When she asks that, she just wants to feel connected to you. She wants to talk, and that's her way of initiating it. Odds are that talking is much more important to her than it is to you. Even in the womb, girls move their mouths much more than boys do.

The other most dreaded question is this: "Honey, why do you love me?" We stumble, mumble, mutter something in response that sounds very much like "Uhhhh, bahh, blub, bub. . . ." How do you put it into words? Here's the secret men need to understand: She wants to hear what makes her special, says Gregory J. P. Godek, author of the best-selling *1001 Ways to Be Romantic* and *Love: The Course They Forgot to Teach You in School.*

"I guarantee you that the reason you fell in love with her was not just because she's a woman," Godek says. "You've known lots of women. They all have the same basic physical attributes, bigger, smaller, in-between." This is the time to hone in on specific attributes. It's the sparkle in her eyes when she looks at a sunset. The way her voice softens when she gets excited. Her mean pot of clam chowder. The way she pretends not to notice when you toss sidelong glances at bikinis.

The point is that only you can answer this question. Think about it—and be ready to dazzle her the next time she asks.

What Women Want

Even the smartest guys wind up shrugging their shoulders and scratching their heads when they're asked what women want from men. "The great question that has never been answered, and which I have not yet been able to answer, despite my 30 years of research into the feminine soul, is 'What does a woman want?'" wrote the great Austrian psychiatrist Sigmund Freud.

It's no wonder this question gave Freud the slip. He may have been an egghead, but he was, after all, a guy—just like the rest of us. So we turned to Ellen Kreidman, Ph.D., a relationship expert and best-selling author of *Light Her Fire* and *The 10-Second Kiss*, for the answer. Here's what she came up with.

It's Not Funny

Women love us when we're funny. A sense of humor is by far the most desired trait that a woman wants to see in a man, says Dr. Paul E. McGhee, president of the Laughter Remedy, a corporate consulting firm that offers programs on humor and laughter in the workplace.

But a sense of humor gone awry is also the thing that can get us in the most trouble. Just because we men think something's funny does *not* mean our women will also be yukking it up. Here is the key, according to licensed professional counselor Carolyn Bushong, author of *The Seven Dumbest Relationship Mistakes Smart People Make*: Do you mock her or someone she cares about? Men, Bushong says, mock each other all the time. It's a way of keeping our egos in check. Women don't share that trait, as any man who has ever said 'Hey, from behind, you look a lot like your mother' can attest.

You can make fun of yourself. In fact, many women appreciate a man who doesn't take himself too seriously. But making fun of her equals disrespect, in her eyes. Yes, it's a double standard. Yes, it makes us think that women lack a sense of humor about themselves. Still, this is a battle you'll always lose. Avoid it.

- She wants to be your first priority.
- She wants you to consider her needs above everyone else's.
- She wants you to think that no other woman comes as close to being perfect for you as she does.
- She wants you to brag about her to your friends and family.
- She wants you to prove your love.
- She wants tender loving care at that time every month when her emotions are ruled by her hormones.

• She needs and expects to have daily reminders of how much you love her.

It's a tall order, to be sure. But the payoff is tremendous—a woman who's there to celebrate your greatest joys and soothe your most crushing disappointments. A woman who looks at you adoringly, even on Saturday morning when you haven't shaved. A woman who will cut you some slack because she trusts you and knows that you're there for her. Oh, and the sex is pretty amazing, too. If that matters.

Who Does the Dishes?

You mow the lawn, mend the porch, trim the shrubs. That's housework, isn't it? It counts, no? Well, yeah, of course it counts. Just not as much as the housework she does.

You know why? Because those manly chores don't compare to the daily drudgery of loading the dirty dishes into the dishwasher, mopping sticky floors, rinsing stinky diapers, and washing load after load of clothes. What commonly have been considered a man's chores have a starting point and a finish, generally celebrated with a cold one. At worst, these are things you do once a week. But the bleak moonscape of housework that has traditionally fallen to women is a monotonous burden.

In 1997, the Gallup Organization asked men and women if husbands did housework. There was an interesting discrepancy. Ninety-seven percent of men flung their hands skyward and said, sure we do. But only 75 percent of women agreed.

Same deal with cooking. Eighty-three percent of husbands claimed they helped with the cooking. Only 63 percent of women agreed. Hey, doesn't the Fourth of July barbecue count for the whole year?

Why Do Women Read Romance Novels?

You say you want to know what a women expects from you. But do you really want to know? To what lengths are you prepared to go? Because if you're stout of heart and stern of character, there are guides that can explicitly spell out what women expect from men.

They're called romance novels.

Now, wait a minute. No part of you is going to shrivel up just because you pick up a book. You don't have to change your name to Zane or Hazard. And you might just learn something.

"Every man might want to read something like this to see what's in women's innermost wild fantasies," says certified sex therapist Wendy Maltz. Women consume romance novels so rapaciously that they comprise half of all paperback novels sold in the United States. There are about 45 million women doing all this buying, of whom 68 percent went to college. Even some full-time, independent,

"What happens in many homes is that she's running around like mad, cleaning everything, and he's there watching television," says Western Kentucky University's Dr. Fred E. Stickle.

Remember, way back at the beginning, when we talked about the sullen silences that can last for days? You've just been introduced to one of the primary reasons. Resentment tends to do that.

Try this compromise, suggests Dr. Stickle. Take a look at the clock, and suggest to your sweetie that you both spend half an hour cleaning up. You take the kitchen, she takes the bathroom. "Then you can both sit down together," he says.

It doesn't end there. You can't just go in and whirl a broom around, either. It has to actually be clean when you're done. Women are far executive-level women admit to reading an average of 14 romances per month.

Not all bodice rippers are created equal, though. Maltz says even her stomach is turned by the smarm in some. A few titles she recommends are Susan Elizabeth Phillips' *Dream a Little Dream*, Elizabeth Lowell's *Winter Fire*, or Susan Johnson's *Blaze*.

"In *Blaze*, the male character is a guy who can skin a buffalo in two hours, yet his kisses are like butterfly wings," says Maltz.

Maybe you can't skin a buffalo, but don't worry: She doesn't actually want you to. It's just the idea that you're a strong, masculine guy. Preferably one who can ravish her with butterfly kisses. "Women don't expect men to be characters from a romance novel, but there are dynamics there that are worth looking into," adds Maltz.

the bedroom will reflect what goes on in the bedroom," says certified sex therapist Wendy Maltz. "Women expect men to know that, and sometimes men are a little perplexed by that fact."

A little? It just doesn't make sense to any male who ever rode a bouncing school bus to erection land. But most women are different. For them, the bus would've needed to have helped them scrub the dishes two days before. That's just the way it is.

Really, it's a good thing that women are wired different than us sexually. There's a lot we can learn from them that takes longer than a five-minute slam dance. By expecting us to go slow, women are actually teaching us wonderful things about intimacy. And that can lead to hotter, more satisfying sex.

"Women also expect men to know something about sex and how it works for them," says Maltz. "And a lot of men don't know."

Or don't care. For example, you've undoubtedly heard that women want to be cuddled after sex. And you want to peacefully drift off. But here's the question: Would you fall asleep if it meant you could rarely have sex in the future? Well, that's what you're doing.

"It makes the woman feel abandoned," explains Maltz. Guess what? She then starts to associate the feeling of being abandoned with having sex with you. How would you feel if you were in her place? Not even an extra-long ride to school would get you going.

Women can be complex, moody, irrational, unpredictable, frustrating, and hormonal creatures. But can you honestly imagine life without them? Their lofty expectations of us are a pittance to pay for a whiff of their perfume, the touch of a hand, a graze of their lips.

So we do what we can. That's the best we can do.

more particular about that, says Joan R. Shapiro, M.D., a Denver psychiatrist and coauthor of *Men: A Translation for Women*. To you, they're insignificant little grains of dust. To her, they're watermelons.

Of course, like any man worth his masculine salt, you need an incentive to get off your butt and help out. Here's a great one.

"Good sex," says Dr. Shapiro. "Foreplay begins in the kitchen." If you're lucky, maybe even on the kitchen table.

Women and Sex

Yes, sad but true, foreplay does begin in the kitchen. And the living room, garage, and shopping mall. "How women are treated out of

What Kids Expect You to Know

How to Be a Gentle Giant

For years, men's role in raising children has been discounted and trod upon. It has sometimes seemed that we were little more than a life-support system for sperm. No more. A spate of recent studies has confirmed what we knew in our hearts all along—dads matter. A lot.

When we're involved in our kids' lives, good things happen. Our daughters are less involved in casual sex. Our sons are less likely to do drugs. Across the board, our children have fewer behavioral problems and a higher sense of themselves when dad is an active parent, explains the University of Colorado Health Sciences Center's Dr. George Hartlaub.

There are numerous reasons for this. First, it may help to realize how our children view us. "We are big and powerful," says Wade F. Horn, Ph.D., president of the National Fatherhood Initiative, a nonprofit community awareness campaign to promote fathers' involvement, and author of *The New Father Book: What Every Man Needs to Know to Be a Good Dad.* "It's both reassuring and a little scary to them."

It's reassuring because you are their protector. You keep away the bad things, from vicious dogs to goblins under the bed. To them, you are strength incarnate.

It's scary because your temperament is the only thing keeping that strength from being used on them. "You re-

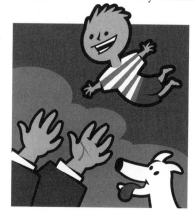

alize, when you're little, that this guy is much bigger than you," Dr. Horn says.

So, you see, this power and strength can serve you well as a father, or it can cause your children to be terrified of you. "It only works if the father combines this natural power with love and affection," says Dr. Horn. Otherwise, you're just a bully.

How do you strike the right balance? Think of your role this way: "One of the most endearing mythic figures to us is the gentle giant," says Dr. Horn. "That's what kids want from their fathers, the gentle giant." That's the guy who stands up big and strong for them, not against them.

Father Knows Best

Now that you know the way your kids see you, let's talk about what they expect from you. Good news—the things that make you a great guy are also the things that make you a great dad. Things like dependability, honesty, your love of fun. Few new skills are required. Here's how to bend those traits to the task of fathering.

Show up for the job. You may have heard that children equate love with time. It's true. "Kids expect us to be there," says Dr. Horn. "Otherwise, how do they learn to count on us? That's the bottom line. Kids want to be able to count on us to be their dads." Your children are very concrete about this. If you loved them, you would be there. If you're not there, it's because you don't love them. Black and white. Cut and dried. The excuses are your problem—they mean nothing to your kids. Divorce, work commitments, alcoholism—that's grown-up stuff; it means nothing to them. Everything else in fatherhood hinges on one simple question: Are you there or not?

Fess up to your mistakes. You're not perfect. Sorry

What Furry Creatures Expect You to Know

So you thought a dog would be a great idea. Man's best friend. Watchdog and companion. A bit of food, a scratch behind the ears every now and then, a squirrel to chase, and he'd be a happy, low-maintenance kind of pal.

Boy, were you wrong.

"What we sometimes do with pets is throw them the occasional emotional Milk-Bone and hope that's enough," says Marty Becker, D.V.M., a veterinarian based in Bonner's Ferry, Idaho, and coauthor of *Chicken Soup for the Pet-Lover's Soul*. But they need so much more. "And if they're given more, they thrive in that environment," he adds.

Take, for example, Dr. Becker's black Labrador retriever, Sirloin. "I don't ever recall a time when I asked Sirloin if he wanted to go out for a walk and he responded, 'You know what, I don't feel like it today,'" he says.

Good news—many of the traits that serve you well as a father will also serve you well as a pet owner. Kids and pets, after all, operate very much on the same wavelength.

"You've basically got two versions of Peter Pan," explains Dr. Becker. "A two-legged version and a four-legged version." Both kids and pets see life through a very similar filter. Both are eternal optimists, live entirely in the present, and don't understand the concept of a stranger. They also tend to lick or drool pretty much equally. But, like kids, your pets have a few expectations of you.

Spend time with them. The big thing is that scarcest of commodities—time. "You have to realize that they have forsaken their own species to be with you," says Dr. Becker. Though pets, by their very nature, would never make you feel this way, you owe them. And that debt is repaid with time.

Play with them. "It's good for their bodies and souls," Dr. Becker says. There is so much joy in their furry bodies that it needs the outlet of play to act as a pressure relief valve. "The urge to play is either bubbling over or just under the surface. It's never not there."

Protect them. Sirloin chased one of Dr. Becker's cats up a tree. In the winter. In a storm. Forty feet off the ground. The kids were begging him to go after the meowing feline. He explained to the kids that, not to worry, as a vet of 20 years, he'd never seen or heard of such a thing as a cat skeleton in a tree. He pointed out that his was only a 20-foot ladder. "Hell, 15 minutes later, guess who's going up the tree," recounts Dr. Becker.

Touch them. "When you rub them or stroke them, there's a positive healing energy that flows from you to them," says Dr. Becker. And back. He says studies have proven that petting an animal mellows you out, lowers your blood pressure, and improves your overall health.

if we're the ones to break it to you, but you're not. And the good news is, your kids don't expect you to be. "So many fathers hear that they need to be good role models and think that means they need to be perfect. That's not what it means at all," says Sal Severe, Ph.D., a school psychologist in Phoenix, president of the Arizona Association of School Psychologists, and author of *How to Behave So Your Children Will, Too!*

So wipe your brow and breathe a sigh of imperfect relief. "What it means is that when we mess up, we take responsibility for it," explains Dr. Severe. Kids understand that we can screw up. What they don't understand is when we blindly stand by mistakes we make. Good dads know they can apologize to their kids and be even more respected because of it.

Be honest. "That's the foundation for trust," says Dr. Severe. It also teaches kids the importance of being honest themselves—a vital characteristic during their teen years when they are confronted with all sorts of potentially unsavory options.

This doesn't mean that you should tell them every dirty detail of your past. "It isn't a matter of saying everything, but what you do say has to be the truth," says Dr. Hartlaub. It also means that when you say you're going to do something, you do it. If you say you're going to be at your kid's T-ball game, you had better be there. "Kids have to be able to count on that," he adds.

Be cool, man. "There's no doubt that kids do things that are worthy of anger, but when you use that anger to get back at them, that's when you do some real damage," says Dr. Severe. Hey, we understand. You get up early, work hard, try to provide for everyone, and then the garbage sits there for two days. It can be an aggravating thing to be a dad. But it's a strong man who keeps his cool when there are flies in the kitchen. "Taking a few minutes is key. Get out of the situation and cool off," recommends Dr. Severe. Deal with yourself, then deal with them.

Take charge. Generations of children grew up fearing those dreaded words "Wait 'til your father gets home." Being the dad has traditionally meant being the main disciplinarian. And despite all of the gender and role changes of the last three decades, that's still usually part of your job description as a dad.

Again, the main thing to keep in mind is to mean what you say and be consistent. If you lay out consequences for an action, you had better follow through. Be clear and specific. Fortunately, we usually don't have much problem holding our kids' toes to the line. "It's easier for us because we're usually not around as much as the mother," says Dr. Hartlaub. Plus, we've generally learned from our own fathers that when the law is laid down, it won't be broken with impunity. We emulate that.

Be playful. This is one of the greatest parts of being a dad. Not only do you get to buy your kids some really nifty toys, you're actually expected to play with them, too. "Kids really expect dads to be playmates, and the nice thing is that we naturally are," says Dr. Horn. "Dads specialize in play." Sure, part of the reason is that we can throw them a zillion feet into the air and generally even catch them. "Kids, on average, actually prefer their dads as playmates. We're more energetic," adds Dr. Horn. "Mothers are softer. Mothers also, even when they play, generally want their kids to learn something. Fathers just want to have a good time."

Safe at Home

Even when fathers take on the task of being the main caregiver, kids thrive, observes Kyle D. Pruett, M.D., a clinical professor of child psychiatry at the Yale Child Study Center. He has found that children raised with dads as the primary caregivers are often active, vital, and vigorous babies, toddlers, preschoolers, and school-age children. And when it comes to solo dads, Dr. Pruett also has made encouraging observations. "Single fathers tend to be open-minded, flexible, and responsive to their children's needs," he says.

Part Two

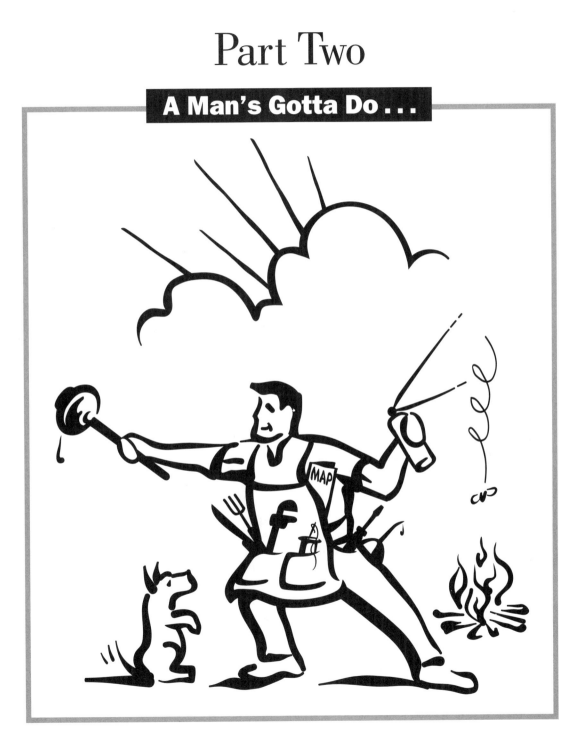

Stand Up to a Bully

The movie *Roxanne* has perhaps one of the best scenes ever showing a bully getting his comeuppance. In it, the character played by Steve Martin has a nose the size of Rhode Island. When a bully tries to provoke him into a bar fight with the lame epithet of "big nose," Martin defuses the tension with a string of 20 jokes at his own expense. A few:

"It's not the size of the nose that's important. It's what's in it that matters."

"When you stop and smell the flowers, are they afraid?"

"Keep that guy away from my cocaine."

The scene illustrates the power of wit in dealing with a bully—the other bar patrons convulse with laughter at Martin's humor, and the bully looks hapless and helpless. Then a less cerebral way of dealing with a bully follows: Martin decks him.

"Bullies are basically looking for power. They're looking for the upper hand on someone," says Howard Knoff, Ph.D., director of the school psychology program at the University of South Florida in Tampa and past president of the National Association of School Psychologists.

The reasons why a guy becomes a bully vary, says Dr. Knoff. He may crave attention. He may have been bullied himself. He could be motivated by revenge. Or, in rare instances, he may even have a physiological or psychological disorder that needs medical or professional attention.

How to Handle a Physical Bully

You have a dilemma. An oaf bearing a striking resemblance to Bluto, the bully nemesis of Popeye for all those years, dares you to fight. Worse, this is in front of your buddies and other people. You don't want to fight—Bluto II has six inches and 60 pounds on you. But you fear losing face by backing down. What do you do?

"In this day and age, if you want to engage in that kind of stuff, you don't know if the guy's armed with a weapon," says Dr. Knoff. "If you want to confront a bully, go for it, but you may ultimately pay a physical price, or a mortal price." Here are some alternatives.

Win the battle of wits. Disarm the pea-brained brute with your verbal virtuosity. Orthopedic surgeon and heavyweight boxer Harold "Hackie" Reitman, of Plantation, Florida, recalls the weigh-in at his first professional fight. His opponent, who was 6 feet 5 inches and 268 pounds, tried to intimidate the 5-foot-10, 215-pound Reitman, who was 38 years old at the time.

The big man shook his fist at Dr. Reitman and threatened to put him in the hospital. "All I did was shake hands and say, 'Well, good luck to you, too, son,'" Dr. Reitman recalls. "I walked away and completely psyched out the guy."

And if you're wondering . . . yes, Dr. Reitman did win the fight, in a second round knockout.

Turn the other cheek. Ignore your tormentor's taunts, suggests Dr. Knoff. Or tell him calmly that you won't be provoked into fighting.

Talk it out. If a guy is itching to fight because he has revenge on his mind, ask him—without raising your voice—to explain what the problem is, says Dr. Knoff. It could be a simple misunderstanding that can be cleared up.

Turn the page. So what happens if the lout is determined to fight you, no matter what? Like we said, make every attempt at resolving the matter peacefully. But if you must fight, turn to Throw a Punch on page 18 for some advice.

How to Handle a Psychological Bully

Not every bully looks like a steroid-crazed NFL lineman. He may weigh 130 pounds and look as menacing as Richard Simmons. "A bully just has to have some element, some characteristic, that enables him to intimidate somebody else," Dr. Knoff says. That element may be a position of power—maybe he's your boss. And his weapon may be mental, not physical, threats. Here's what you can do about it.

Keep your cool. Don't respond to a bully's tirade angrily or defensively, advises James Campbell Quick, Ph.D., professor of organizational behavior at the University of Texas at Arlington and editor of the *Journal of Occupational Health Psychology*. He tells the story of a bullying boss for whom his grandfather once worked. One day, after one of his rants, the boss asked granddad if he ever got mad. "I don't need to; you get angry enough for both of us," granddad replied evenly.

"He didn't get angry. He didn't get hostile. He simply asserted himself," says Dr. Quick. At the same time, he legitimized his boss's feelings: "You get angry a lot, I understand that. But you're not going to push me around." The boss never harangued him again.

Make eye contact. "What you're doing nonverbally is according him power and acknowledging him. 'You are important, I'm paying attention to you,'" says Dr. Quick. Looking the bully in the eye and speaking calmly to him is a way to stand up to him in a nonconfrontational manner and calm him down. He will be less likely to bully you in the future, and you may even gain his respect, says Dr. Quick.

Bully Boys

A dad's dilemma: What do you do if your son is being picked on by a bully? Don't exhort him to give the bully a taste of his own medicine. "You may be setting your kid up for a very dangerous situation," says the University of South Florida's Dr. Howard Knoff, who consults with schools on how to deal with bullies.

What about martial arts training for your boy? "If parents are doing this for the kid's self-protection, it's probably not a good idea. It's reinforcing or encouraging a kid to use violence as a way to solve a problem. In most situations, that's not going to solve the problem," says Dr. Knoff.

Instead, notify school administrators if your son is being bullied on an ongoing basis, and get assurances that they will handle the matter confidentially, says Dr. Knoff. They may call in the parents of both boys to try to get at the root of the problem.

If your son is being bullied in grade school, speak to the bully's teacher rather than school administrators, suggests Dr. Knoff. "In elementary school, the teacher is going to have a stronger handle on it," he says. "The teachers know the kids a little bit more intimately."

Ask for suggestions. If your boss is berating you over a decision you made, calmly ask him what he would have had you do instead, Dr. Quick suggests. This puts the responsibility on him to tell you specifically what he really wants done.

Praise him. If your bully boss does something genuinely worthy of praise, compliment him privately. It could transform your relationship, Dr. Quick says.

Throw a Punch

We don't know whether or not it is man's basic nature to be violent. Some guys who profess to abhor fighting fight nonetheless.

"You know I hate fighting," Muhammad Ali once said. "If I knew how to make a living some other way, I would."

Harold "Hackie" Reitman, M.D., knows how to make a living some other way. He's a successful orthopedic surgeon. But at age 38, he launched a second career—professional boxer. This heavyweight has sparred with 32 world champions and continues to fight professionally well into his late forties. Yet he says with all sincerity, "I don't condone violence. Do everything you can to avoid getting into a fight."

Regardless of whether your own temperament is wild or mild, there may come a time when you simply can't avoid a fight no matter how hard you try. You lie on your back and bare your throat to your antagonist. You offer him your wallet and your watch as a peace offering. Hell, you even compliment him on his pierced tongue and hairy knuckles. And still he wants to provide you with the gift of a new orifice. It can be handy, in these circumstances, to know some fighting basics.

Or you may just want to try boxing in the gym. It's a superb workout. Either way, here are the basics to get you started.

Don't be a square. Your weight must be distributed evenly on both feet in order to deliver a powerful punch, says Angelo Dundee, the legendary trainer who instructed 15 world champions, including Muhammad Ali, George Foreman, Sugar Ray Leonard, and Jimmy Ellis, on the nuances of pugilism. "Don't stand in a square position," Dundee advises. "The left foot must be in front and the right foot must be in back if you're right-handed, and if you're left-handed, the opposite. And turn your body somewhat sideways. You don't stand square because you're giving a bigger target of yourself."

Your feet should be spread wide enough that you don't get them tangled. How wide depends on your height and what feels comfortable, Dundee says. "You have to have your feet in position so you can go forward or go back," he says. "If you throw a right-handed punch, your right or rear foot should not leave the ground," Dundee says. Instead, you swivel on the ball of your foot.

Put your weight behind it. As you pivot on your rear foot, swivel your hips, torso, and the shoulder of your punching arm as your weight moves forward, generating torque and power. "Your power does not come from your arm," says Dr. Reitman, who is a former Golden Gloves champion. "The idea is to use your leverage to get your whole body weight behind the punch. When you see these big muscle-bound fighters, they usually can't break an egg because they're just doing what we call arm punching. They're not using their whole body to deliver the punch."

Bend your knees. When you hit somebody, your knees should be slightly bent. "It gives you more leverage," Dundee says.

Delivering the Punch Line

Jab first. Don't lead with your right hand if you are right-handed, or your left if you're left-handed, Dundee advises. Jab with your other hand. This does two things. It creates openings for delivering the big blows, and it helps you determine the distance to your opponent and whether you need to move in closer to make a good punch. "If you get a fighter who can't jab, I'll show you a loser," Dundee says.

When throwing a left jab, step forward slightly with your left foot and extend your arm, says Dr. Reitman. The punch should be short and straight.

Keep your hands and elbows in close. When you're setting up to hit a guy, your arms should be in close to your body. This helps you throw straighter punches and protect your own head and body, Dr. Reitman says.

Does Size Really Matter?

Students of the sweet science of boxing say that technique is more important than raw power or sheer size when trying to deliver a powerful punch.

Rocky Marciano would seem to prove their point.

The Rock was one of the most prolific heavyweight knockout artists of all time. He won all 49 of his fights, 43 either by knockout or the referee stopping the bout. Yet Marciano was less than six feet tall and weighed only 185 pounds.

"If your arms are outside of your body, you don't have the same snap," Dundee adds.

Extend your arm. As you throw a punch, your arm should be extended all the way out, Dundee says. The punch ought to be thrown at about the height of your own jawline.

When you bring your arm back, keep it at about that height. If you drop your punching hand, your adversary can respond with a blow of his own in the opening you have created, Dr. Reitman says. Most important, a good punch needs to be straight and true. One of the biggest mistakes amateurs make is to throw wide, sweeping punches, he says.

Set   Throw

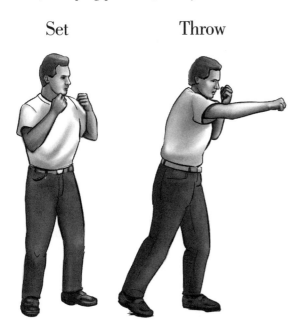

Follow through. For maximum impact, drive your fist forward after impact. "You're going through the object," Dr. Reitman says. "You're not stopping at the guy's head."

Do the slide. Even if the other guy grabs you and gets you in a clinch, you can deliver a punishing punch, Dundee says. If you're right-handed, just slide to the right, then nail him. Mike Tyson was one of the best at this, Dundee adds.

Twist your fist. When you start to throw a punch, you most likely are holding your fist with the thumb side facing up. As you deliver a blow, rotate your fist so the palm faces down, Dundee says. And make sure to tuck your thumb under your fingers to avoid injury, he adds.

Pick your spots. If your technique is good, any punch you throw can hurt an opponent. But some places hurt more than others. "The temple, if you can throw it without looping it, is a particularly vulnerable place," Dr. Reitman says. "A straight jab to the bridge of the nose or a blow to the jaw can be pretty effective as well."

Don't hold back. If you have to duke it out with somebody, remember that it's not going to be a matter of pacing yourself. A fight is exhausting, especially if you haven't trained for it. "It's not going to be a long, drawn-out affair because civilians can't go more than a minute," Dr. Reitman says. "If you are unfortunate enough to be forced into a fight, make it quick."

Find Your Way

Tim Cahill has been horseback riding in Mongolia. He's hung out with diamond miners at a squalid camp in Venezuela. Heck, he has even tumbled into a group of mountain gorillas in Rwanda. And after visiting about 75 countries in 20 years, Cahill, an editor-at-large for *Outside* magazine in Santa Fe, New Mexico, has been lost. Lots of times. But losing your way, he says, can enhance your travels, rather than ruin them.

"Getting lost is one of the privileges of traveling," says Cahill, who has written several adventure travel books, including *Pass the Butterworms: Remote Journeys Oddly Rendered.* "Savor it when you get lost."

The best way to find your way home again is simply to ask for directions, says Cahill. He realizes some guys would rather spend time in a Turkish prison than ask for help, but Cahill says that there is plenty of upside to piping up.

"In my years of professional traveling, I've found that most strangers are kind, and the most noteworthy, amusing, and inspirational experiences I've had have come when I've been lost," Cahill says. "I kind of like getting lost."

Asking a native for help when you're lost has other benefits besides getting you pointed in the right direction, according to Cahill. "Having to ask directions is a perfectly good way to strike up a conversation," he says. In some places, "there's this sort of thing where a guy suddenly says, 'I have to show you my city.' He becomes your best friend on Earth for maybe two to three hours, and you go out and have a great time together. He takes you to his favorite places, walking you back to where you started—and then you never see the guy again."

If, however, you still stubbornly refuse to ask for directions, here are a few things you can do to try to minimize trouble, Cahill says.

Use a compass. Cahill wears a watch with a compass. "I've found that it's very helpful," he says. Or you can buy a compass that straps on to your other wrist.

Stay calm. You'll only have more trouble figuring out where you are when you're flustered, Cahill says.

Don't get drunk in unfamiliar places. "If you have your wits about you, presumably you're not going to wander into a rough part of the city," Cahill says.

Maps and Legends

Cahill's advice is valuable if you're dazed and confused in Baghdad or Rangoon, but what if your typical vacation takes you only to the balmy beaches of Fort Lauderdale or the steep streets of San Francisco?

First, learn some basic map-reading skills. "Fewer people than you might expect know how to read a map effectively," says Jerry Cheske, director of public relations at the AAA (American Automobile Association) National Office in Heathrow, Florida.

Here are a few things that can make reading a map at least somewhat easier than deciphering hieroglyphics.

Pick a map drawn to the proper scale. The smaller the number after the colon, the greater the detail of the map. A 1:10,000 scale would be good for hiking, while a scale of 1:25,000 would show many details of a large city, say map makers Rand McNally. A scale of 1:500,000 or 1:1,000,000 would do when planning a long driving trip.

Place the map in the same direction you are facing. If you're walking or driving south, for example, align the map in that direction. "It can help some people," says Cheske. "You need to have a feel for where you're standing and where you're facing in relation to the map."

Read the legend. If guys would take a minute to read a map's legend, many map mysteries would be solved. On one map, for example, the legend might tell you that a thick red line is a multi-lane, divided road—typically an interstate or similar highway. A fat orange line is a toll road, such as a turnpike. Thin gray lines are dirt roads, and so on. The color scheme may change from map to map—that's one more reason why you need to read the legend.

Get specific. If map reading is not your forte, get step-by-step directions when possible. Some people understand specific instructions—drive 25 miles on Interstate 95, exit west on Commercial Boulevard, then turn right on Dixie Highway—more easily than trying to deduce the same information from a map, says Cheske.

Even if you're a modern-day Meriwether Lewis, specific instructions won't solve all your travel travails. Many city streets have two names, or a name and a route number. "Most good maps should show both," Cheske says.

Getting Back on Track

When you do get lost, Cheske says guys need to avoid muddling ahead, turning a minor glitch into a nerve-frazzling fiasco. "You may need to think in terms of damage control and not getting more lost. The key is to correct the problem as soon as possible," he says. "That means pulling over and asking for directions, or pulling out a map and figuring out just where you are."

Both Cheske and Cahill caution that men need to be a bit skeptical about directions they receive from somebody. "I don't think you can assume that the person is giving you gospel information," says Cheske. "You may want to check it against your own feelings after reading a map." If you don't have a map, ask more than one person for directions to see if you get a consensus opinion, adds Cahill.

Cheske admits that even he is reluctant to seek help. "I think men have a feeling that they have an innate sense of navigation," he says. "It's a feeling of accomplishment when

Fightin' Words

Getting lost often means ending up in a neighborhood so rough even the women look like they can kick your butt. It's especially unsettling in a foreign country, where because of the color of your skin or the way you're dressed, you can't possibly blend in.

What to do? Buy a local newspaper or magazine, and carry it with you everywhere, advises Tim Cahill, an editor-at-large for *Outside* magazine. "You may be an obvious foreigner. But people look at you with the local paper and they figure that you must live here. You don't look like such an immediate mark," he says.

If a local no-neck is wise to your guise and starts to hassle you, your periodical can still save your salsa, points out Cahill. "If you roll it sideways very tightly, it's an incredibly destructive weapon," he says. "You hit the person with the end of the thing. It has the effect of a lead pipe."

Here's the part we like best of all. "If worse came to worst and you're arrested, you don't have a weapon on you," Cahill notes. "You just have a magazine."

Now that's the power of the press.

you can handle the trip, and there is a certain feeling of adventure—'we're heading north still, we're okay.' "

For those who want the journey made simple, however, there is one other option, says Cheske. You can buy a car—or have yours equipped—with a satellite navigation system. This technology enables you to tell a computer where you are and where you want to go. The system will describe available options, then tell you if you miss a turn and how to recalculate your route if you do.

"These systems are amazingly accurate," Cheske says.

Choose and Train a Dog

Is your dog so dense he flunked obedience school? Don't despair. "I have never seen a dog that could not learn simple remedial tasks," says Amy Ammen, a Milwaukee dog trainer and author of three books, including *Dog Training for a Happy, Healthy Pet.*

Why bother? "Not only does it make him a much more enjoyable pet for you and anyone who might have to take care of him, but dogs are happier and more confident when they've been through training," Ammen says.

Picking the Right Pup

Here are some things to consider when choosing a dog.

Size up your lifestyle. Even a big dog can adapt to small living quarters, depending on his owner's lifestyle, says Quenten London, an animal behaviorist at the National Institute of Dog Training in Los Angeles. A Dalmatian, for example, needs vigorous exercise, but an apartment dweller can provide this by going for walks or runs with the dog every day. "It's not the space, it's your lifestyle," London says.

Take his temperament. If you have a small child, you don't want an aggressive dog. Some breeds tend to be more combative, such as Akitas, cocker spaniels, Rottweilers, and even some smaller breeds, London says. And other breeds, such as the retrievers, can be especially gentle. But remember that it's not the breed, but the breeding, that will determine how your dog will behave.

When you're attempting to determine a puppy's temperament, try pulling gently on his tail or his jowls and pressing gently on his paws. If he doesn't get riled, you may have found a good dog for kids, London says.

Dogs should be supervised with children until the dogs are at least nine months old, Ammen says. Children also need supervision with dogs—to a considerably older age that varies, but it's usually around 7 to 10 years of age, she says.

Let him age. If you buy a puppy, make sure he's at least seven weeks old, Ammen says. That's enough time for the critter to interact with his mom and littermates so that he knows how to behave around other dogs when he becomes older.

Don't miss demeanor. A puppy should appear alert and enjoy being with people and his littermates. If he cowers or runs for cover at the slightest noise, he probably is easily stressed, Ammen says.

Search for a breeder apart. Ask kennel clubs for the names of reputable breeders, Ammen suggests. Ask to meet the pup's parents, and only buy a dog from a breeder who provides a guarantee concerning the animal's health and temperament.

Animal shelters also are a good place to find dogs—and they're far cheaper. "If someone is willing to do the training, they can end up with a real champ," Ammen says. While you can find purebred dogs at animal shelters, London and Ammen both stress that mixed breeds also make terrific pets. Some animal shelters can provide a history on an animal.

Basic Training

You needn't prepare your new pet for a drill at the Westminster Dog Show in order to make him a more cultured creature in the canine world. Here's how to turn your mutt into a top dog.

Be consistent. Don't scold your dog for begging at the table one time, then slip him a morsel the next night, Ammen says. Lack of consistency contributes to his misbehavior, she says.

Start early. You can begin teaching

simple commands such as sit, down, and come to a puppy as soon as you bring him home, Ammen says. By four months of age, he should comprehend what you're saying.

Keep it brief. Dogs have short attention spans. And that's especially true of puppies. Limit your training time to one or two 10-minute sessions a day if he's less than four months old, Ammen suggests. A dog older than that may stay focused for 30 minutes at a time. "If you are working on something the dog has an aptitude for, you may find that you can train that dog far longer," Ammen says.

Have a release word. "There should be a formal way he is told that you're all done," Ammen says. A touch under the dog's chin while you say "okay" is one possible release method. If you prefer, no word at all is necessary. Pointers in the field won't go off point unless they receive a touch on the head or hindquarters by their owners, Ammen says.

Be kind and gentle. "You never want to hit your dog," London says. "You never want to yell at your dog. It creates fear and lack of trust. Without trust, the dog won't do what you ask him to."

Use rewards. Try using small treats to get the puppy's attention, London says. Give a tiny morsel, about the size of a pea, to a puppy before you begin a training session in order to get his attention. When he does a command correctly, reward him with another, and always praise him. Eventually, wean him off the treats, when you are confident that he understands your commands.

Just say no. When correcting your dog, don't use his name when you say "no," advises London. "Then he won't trust you when you call him," he says. Just say "no" not, "No, Rex."

House Rules

No training is as urgent as housebreaking a new dog—especially if you're the one who has to clean up after him. Here's what you need to know.

Be on schedule. Try to provide food and water to your pup as well as go for walks at about the same time every day, suggests Quenten London of the National Institute of Dog Training. While you're at work, see if somebody can let him out briefly during the day. Make his last meal no later than 5:30 P.M., and be sure to take him outside before you go to bed—always praising him if he relieves himself there.

Boycott the news. Don't place newspapers on the floor, London advises. That tactic teaches a dog to relieve himself only indoors.

Catch him in the act. If you catch your dog relieving himself in the house, say "no" and carry him outside in midstream. Praise him if he finishes in the yard, says London. Don't scold the dog after the fact. He won't know what he has done wrong.

Remove odors. When your dog does go on the floor, use a powerful neutralizer to clean up, London says. If any hint of the odor remains, the dog will go in that same area again.

Isolate him. When you can't supervise your pup, and when you go to bed at night, place him in a wire crate. This serves as his den, and dogs don't want to foul their dens, explains London.

Be terse. Use simple one-word commands, London says. Say "stay" rather than "stay there" and "Rex, come" instead of "come here," for example. Only use the dog's name for "heel" and "come" commands.

Fix a Leaky Faucet

If you've thumbed your way to this chapter because it's 3:00 in the morning and that dripping faucet is keeping you up, don't sweat it. Grab a washcloth and toss it under the tap. It'll muffle the noise until daybreak. Go back to bed—we'll meet up here again in the morning.

Okay, we're back. You awake? Ready to go to work? All right, let's tweak that leak and stop that drop. Chances are, you have one of two types of faucets. The most common taps are either a two-handled compression faucet or a single-handle rotating ball faucet, says Alain G. Giroux, a licensed plumber in Ottawa, Ontario. Let's start with the first one.

The Compression Faucet

It's called a compression faucet because that's what it does. There's a handle for the hot water and one for the cold. When you turn them off, they screw downward and compress a rubber washer against the supply hole. When that washer wears thin, it starts to leak. These are the most common style of faucets and also the easiest to repair. Here are the steps Giroux recommends.

Turn off the water supply. Sounds like a no-brainer, but Giroux says he has seen plenty of people forget. "And, bam, the water hits the wall, ceiling, dog, and cat," he says. Save the floods for Noah and look under the sink for two shut-off valves. If there aren't any, trace the pipes back to the nearest ones. Turn the taps on before you start working to ensure that the supply is off.

Doff your cap. Pry the cap off the top of each handle. You'll see a screw underneath holding the handle to the stem assembly. Unscrew it and lift the handle off.

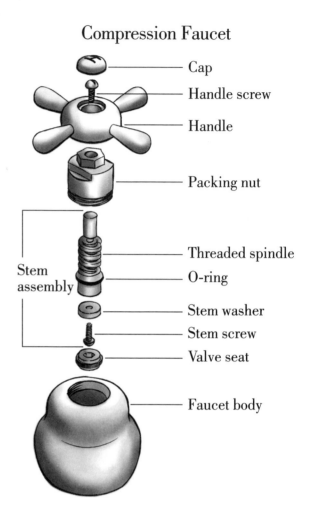

Compression Faucet

- Cap
- Handle screw
- Handle
- Packing nut
- Stem assembly
- Threaded spindle
- O-ring
- Stem washer
- Stem screw
- Valve seat
- Faucet body

Stem the tide. Take an adjustable wrench and fit it to the hexagonal packing nut that holds the stem to the faucet body. Unscrew it counterclockwise and lift the stem out. You'll see two rubber pieces. One is an O-ring that looks like a thick, circular rubber band. The other is the washer on the bottom of the stem. It's held on with a screw; the O-ring just hugs on to the stem. Take them both off and set them aside.

Take a seat. While you're at it, you'll probably want to change the valve seat as well. It's the metal ring that the washer presses against. When a washer first begins to wear out, you can stop the faucet from dripping by cranking down harder on the tap. You probably kept doing that until it just didn't work anymore. Well, what you did was grind the metal of the stem against the metal of the valve seat, scratching and gouging the valve seat to the point that—even with a new washer—it probably won't seal properly.

Replace the worn parts. Find a set of Allen wrenches and remove the valve seat. It usually takes a ⅜-inch wrench. Insert the end down into the hole and turn counterclockwise. Take the valve seat, the O-ring, and the washer down to the hardware store and buy identical replacements. Reassemble the faucet by reversing what you did to take it apart. Make sure you screw the washer on tightly, or it will flap like a chicken passing a KFC when the water rushes by it. Oh, and turn the water back on.

The Ball Faucet

A ball faucet is a single-handle tap, the kind where you move it to the left for hot and to the right for cold. One common make is Delta. But like a gelding, not all single-handle taps have a ball. If your faucet has a round cap just under the handle, it's probably a rotating ball fixture. Here's how to replace the innards, according to Giroux.

Handle the problem right. Turn off the water supply. Find a small Allen wrench to fit the setscrew near the front and bottom of the handle. Loosen it and remove the handle.

Be a man of the cloth. Use a large pair of pliers and turn the rounded cap counterclockwise to remove it. If you wrap the chromed cap with a cloth first, the pliers won't scratch it.

Make the cam scram. Take out the plastic cam, rubber cam seal, and ball. Look down into the hollow and use a small screwdriver to pull out the two little rubber seals and the springs beneath them.

Be sure the kit fits. Take the whole works down to the hardware store and get a replacement kit to match. Replace the guts in

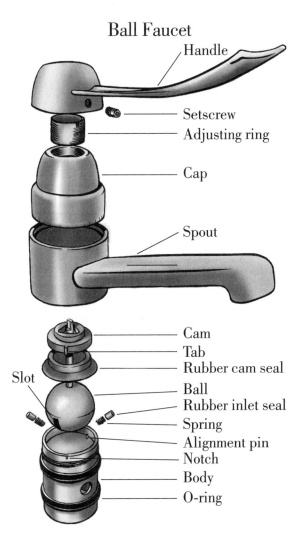

Ball Faucet

Handle
Setscrew
Adjusting ring
Cap
Spout

Cam
Tab
Rubber cam seal
Slot
Ball
Rubber inlet seal
Spring
Alignment pin
Notch
Body
O-ring

the order you took them out. The new ball will have an alignment groove that fits over a pin in the hollow it came from. Make sure it matches up.

Make adjustments. Before you put the handle back on, turn on the water supply. There's a small adjusting ring on the top of the rounded cap that regulates how tightly the ball gets pushed into the rubber seals. If the faucet is leaking, use the little tool you got in the replacement kit to tighten the adjusting ring. Do it just enough to stop the leaking. Put the handle back on.

Clean a Carpet Stain

Upset about a little cat puke on your rug? Well, cry us a river. When Neal A. Smither goes in to clean a carpet, he's decked out in a full body suit, gloves, boots, and an oxygen mask.

See, Smither is president of Crime Scene Cleaners, a San Francisco Bay–area company that specializes in picking up and putting right homes and businesses after murders, suicides, and accidental deaths. His company goes into places where only the most stern of stomach dare tread. Still, it's just another day at work for Smither. "When I smell decomposition, that's really the smell of job security to me," he says.

The point? Whatever is on your carpet could be worse. With that in mind, here are some smart strategies to get the splat out of your mat, courtesy of Smither and Michael Hilton, technical associate in cleaning and maintenance at the Carpet and Rug Institute in Dalton, Georgia.

Act quickly. Most spills can be removed if you deal with them right away. The longer you wait, the more they set.

Blot the spot. Get a dry, white, absorbent towel or paper towel. No patterns or colors, please. Colors in the towels could transfer to the carpet. Press down gently and soak up the spill.

Don't scrub, Bub. Scrubbing instead of blotting can distort the pile of the carpet. Just keep blotting until the area is dry, Hilton says. If it's a semi-solid like dog poop, get a spoon and gently scrape it up. (Note: Don't put the spoon back in the silverware drawer when you're done.)

Water it down. Once you've finished blotting, remove any residual staining with a liquid. If in doubt, use water. "It's the universal solvent," says Hilton. Dampen a clean, white cloth and work in gently from the edges of the stain. Keep blotting, absorbing as much as possible, and repeat until clean. It may take a couple of treatments, so don't get frustrated.

Polish it up. Nail polish remover is especially effective on oil-based stains. Acetone or non-acetone will work, but non-acetone is better, according to Hilton. Non-acetone contains amyl acetate or ethyl acetate, which are paint, oil, and grease removers. Whichever type you use, never pour it directly on your carpet. Instead, pour some on a rag and use it to blot as directed above. Make sure you blot afterwards with lukewarm water, unless it's a blood stain, in which case you should use cold. Also, never saturate your backing (the underside of a carpet) with the nail polish remover since the backing is latex and nail polish remover may cause it to break down.

Say bye to blood. The best way to keep from having to clean up blood spills is to simply not shoot or stab anybody. "That's really the ideal way to avoid it," says Smither. But if you have a minor accident and get some blood on the carpet, Smither recommends a product called Simple Green, an all-purpose cleaner. He has seen it work on the most gruesome of stains. First test it on a small piece of your carpet because its green color may discolor your carpeting. If it tests okay, apply some to a rag. Then, working from the inside of the stain outwards, rub very lightly to remove it. When you're through, go back over the spot using a water-dampened rag.

Leave the solids solid. If it's something like baby powder, never put any liquid on it. You'll turn it into a paste. Just run the vacuum over any solid spill until it's gone.

Plan ahead. Some events just lend themselves to spills. "If you have a big Super Bowl party going and the beer's spilling, you can't just stop the party," says Hilton. Instead, stock up on some dry carpet-cleaning powder such as Host or Capture, which are available at vacuum and flooring stores. Sprinkle it on the beer. It can then even sit overnight until you're sober enough to clean it up in the morning.

Unstop a Toilet

It's a strange thing. If a man retches, gags, coughs, and whines enough, he can often get out of changing a diaper. Why then is it so unquestionably his job when the toilet gets plugged up? It's the same stuff, just a different location.

Whatever the philosophical reasons, someone has lightened their load at your expense, and there's an unpleasant task ahead. The first thing you'll need is a way to deal with the smell. Licensed plumber Alain G. Giroux has been known to eat his lunch while elbow-deep in a blocked toilet. He offers these tips.

Breathe through your mouth. Bypass your olfactory system altogether.

Light some matches. The sulfuric smell does a good job of canceling out other odors.

Wet a rag and tie it around your face. A wet rag does a better job of filtering out bad smells than a dry one, according to Giroux.

Choose Your Weapons

If it's a relatively loose blockage, you should be okay with just a plunger. Giroux says the funnel-cup plungers work best. Those are the ones with the added piece extending off the bottom of the rubber cup. No matter what type of plunger you use, if the rubber is stiff and old, he recommends running it under hot water for a minute. That will soften the rubber and make a better seal. If you're feeling particularly dainty, feel free to go ahead and put on a pair of rubber gloves, too. Then follow these steps, Giroux says.

Take the plunge. Place the plunger in the bowl and give the blockage three hard shots. Check to see if the water level drops. If it

does, try flushing. If not, put the plunger back and give it four or five fast, shallow thrusts, keeping the plunger in contact with the bowl throughout.

Unleash the auger. If plunging doesn't work, try a closet auger. Available at most hardware stores, it's a cablelike device that rotates through the blockage. Giroux stresses that you should only use the auger if you know the blockage is caused by human waste and toilet paper. If it's something else, the auger will push it into the main and cause a blockage there.

Feed the auger into the hole until it stops. Then lock the handle with the thumbscrew and turn it clockwise. Slowly withdraw the cable. With luck, you've hooked the blockage and pulled it out.

Know when to call a pro. If, after repeated efforts, the clog won't clear, you probably have a blocked main or a more solid obstruction in the drain. The toilet will have to come off. Call a plumber.

Keep It Flowing

Chances are, you don't want to go through this on a regular basis. Then you should know the most common causes of a blocked toilet. Aside from regular human waste, these are the things that Giroux most often sees clogging a john.

Dental floss. "It's like fish line. You can't break it," he says. It snags in the drain and catches the stuff that follows.

Q-tips. "A Q-tip is about 3 inches. A drain hole is 2½." Do the math.

Condoms. They can snag, and the flowing water can fill them like a balloon. Sure, it sounds like fun. But trust us—it's not.

Toothbrushes. "I don't know how they get in there so often," admits Giroux. "Some people must brush their teeth in the bowls, and when the seats hit them on their heads, they drop their brushes."

Unclog a Drain

One definition of the word *sink* is "a place where vice, corruption, or evil collects." So *that* is what's under that murky pool of water standing in your basin. Arm yourself, Don Johnson, it's time to play vice squad.

Your weapons of choice will be a plunger, a bucket, and a small towel. If you have a funnel-cup plunger, the one with the extra lip that hangs down, tuck it back up so the bottom is flat. If the rubber is stiff, run it under hot water for a minute to make it pliable, says licensed plumber Alain G. Giroux.

If you're thinking about taking the easy way out by buying some industrial strength drain opener and mixing yourself a drain cocktail, stop. Right now. Those caustic substances only work if there's some flow of water through the drain. If it's plugged tight, Drano and its cousins will just sit in the sink, and you'll find out that stainless steel doesn't live up to its name. Porcelain will also discolor and the drain opener will dissolve the plastic seals in your pipes. If you've already taken this route with these results, call a plumber and warn him that there's drain opener lurking in your sink.

Here is Giroux's alternate battle plan.

Take a pop. If you're in the bathroom, remove the pop-up stopper. Most stoppers lift straight out; some you may have to turn first. If there's hair and other nasty stuff hanging on to it, pull it off. That may be all that's blocking the sink. If you're in a double-basin kitchen sink, put the plug in the sink you're not working on.

Plug the overflow. If the sink has an overflow hole near the top of the basin, wet the towel and stuff it in so you won't dissipate the force of the plunger. If the sink has no overflow, keep the towel handy to mop your brow and pretend that you're working hard.

Man the bucket brigade. Put your bucket under the drainpipes below the sink. If there isn't enough water already, fill the sink up to at least four inches. Take your plunger and give the drain four or five rapid shots, concentrating more on speed than strength. "If you pump too hard, it'll disconnect the drainpipes," warns Giroux. That's why you put the bucket under there—just in case.

Check, please. Stand back and check the water level. If it clears, run hot water into the drain for at least a minute to wash down any remaining crud. Call it a day.

Open your trap. If the sink is still clogged, you'll have to remove the P-trap—the P-shaped pipe directly below the sink. To do this, loosen both slip nuts on either side of the curved trap with groove-joint pliers or a wrench. Yes, the water in the pipe will trickle out, but that's why you have the bucket underneath. Take a wire coat hanger, straighten it, and bend a hook in one end. Use the hook to fish out whatever is blocking the trap. Reassemble the drain.

If that didn't do the trick, you probably have a blockage farther back in the pipe in the wall. It's time to call a plumber.

Pipe Down

Most blockages can be avoided with a little foresight, Giroux says. Always use a strainer over the drain in the kitchen, no matter how tempting it may be to wedge those niblets down the pipe. And never pour grease down the drain. Even if it clears the trap, it will solidify in the main and cause big problems down the road.

Most blockages build up over time, says Giroux. He suggests this trick to keep your sink free-flowing: Once a week, fill the sink half-full with hot water (preferably boiling). Add four tablespoons of baking soda and about one-half cup of vinegar to the water. Use a pair of pliers to pull the plug so you don't burn your fingers. After the solution drains, run the hot water for another minute or so. Brag to your friends about how clean the inside of your pipes are.

Reset a Pilot Light

If you're greeted by an icy cold blast of water in your morning shower, the usual suspect is the pilot light on the water heater. Before you try to relight it yourself, a word of caution: You'll get a whiff of gas as you light the pilot light, but you shouldn't be able to smell it before or after. If you do, shut off the gas. Most units can be shut off at the control knob on the water heater, in the area of the thermostat. Otherwise, you can shut off the fuel by flipping the valve on the fuel line, several feet from the water heater. (To turn it off, flip the handle so it points perpendicular to the pipe.)

Don't switch anything electrical on or off. Clear out of the house—leaving the doors open—and call the gas company from a neighboring phone. Even the small sparks in a telephone can ignite heavy concentrations of gas, says Ross Willis, a spokesman for the Atlanta Gas Light Company based in Atlanta.

Even if you don't smell gas but you feel uncomfortable working with gas appliances, go ahead and call a professional, adds Willis.

Here are some common causes of a doused pilot light.

- The fuel supply is off. If you have propane, check to see if your tank has juice. If not, pay your bill and sheepishly relight the pilot. If you have natural gas, check to see if other gas appliances are working, advises Willis. If not, get on the blower to the gas company and tell them.
- The doggone kids. The main gas valve switch is designed to have easy access in case of emergency, says Willis. "But boys will be boys," he adds. Check to make sure a child didn't shut it off.
- A bad thermocouple. Thermocouples are safety features that shut down the flow of gas if the pilot light is extinguished. This prevents gas from building up in the house. When one conks out, it'll take the pilot with it. If the pilot won't relight, it's probably a thermocouple. Call a repairman.

Now it's time to fire that baby back up. Here's how, according to Willis and the safety experts at Atlanta Gas Light Company.

- Open the windows, doors, and vents in the room to provide ventilation.
- Remove the access panel at the bottom of the heater. Sometimes there's another one covering the pilot. Take that off, too.
- Turn the gas control knob (it's usually red) to "off" and wait a minimum of five minutes to allow any gas in the pipes to be cleared. Then turn the gas control knob to "pilot."
- Ignite a long fireplace match or a gas grill lighter with a long nose, and hold it near the tip of the pilot. When your flame is stable, press the red pilot ignition button and hold. If there's no button, try pushing on the gas control knob. It serves a dual purpose on some heaters.
- After the flame gets going, keep the button pressed in for about a minute, and then slowly release it. The pilot should stay lit.
- After noting the setting of the thermostat (the large dial in front of the control), turn it to the lowest setting. This is done to prevent starting out with an overload of fuel. You can now turn the gas control knob back to "on."
- If the pilot stays on, put the access panels back in place. Now you are in a safer position to return the thermostat dial to its previous setting, Willis says.
- So that you can access them the next time, tape instructions on the back of the water heater—either the ones that came with the appliance or a copy of this chapter. If the pilot won't light or flickers back out, you have more serious woes and probably need a pro. Let your fingers do the walking.

Replace a Button

Sir Isaac Newton once said that science requires that you replace many buttons.

Well, he didn't really put it in those exact words, but consider this: According to the National Center for Health Statistics, the number of overweight adults increased from 26 to 35 percent between 1976 and 1994. And Newton's third law of motion says that for every action there is an equal and opposite re-action. Hence, more popped buttons. It's simple science.

A Stitch in Time

Turning from Newton's law to Murphy's, you probably lost your button at the most inconvenient time. Fear not, there's help all around you. Most hotels have emergency sewing repair kits at the front counter. Also, check the vending machines at interstate service plazas and at airports; they often sell needles and thread. Otherwise, pick up a repair kit at most drugstores, department stores, or even supermarkets.

For shirts, you can usually find a replacement button down on the shirttails. Same with good quality pants, except the extra buttons are attached to the inside of the belt area. Once you have a needle, thread, and a new button, it's time to start stitching. Here's how, according to Judith Kronmeyer, a retired home economics teacher in Waretown, New Jersey, and a former home economist for *Good Housekeeping* magazine.

Get thready. It may be easier for a camel to go through the eye of a needle than for a rich man to enter the kingdom of God, but it's none too easy for a slender sliver of thread, either. Start by cutting the tip of the thread with scissors to give it an even, sharp point. Then give the tip a lick and a spit to keep it from unraveling.

Contrast it. Use a piece of white paper as a background to your needle and thread. This gives you some contrast to work with and makes it easier to see the eye of the needle. Glide the thread through. If you miss a few times and start to fray the end, recut the thread and start over.

Stretch it. Pull through about 36 inches of thread. Double it over and pull the needle to the center of the length. Knot the two free ends together so that you have about 18 inches of doubled-over thread.

Sew it. Start from the back and pull the thread through where you want to sew on the button, Kronmeyer says. Drop your button down over the needle through one of the holes. You need to leave some space between the button and the fabric. Kronmeyer suggests placing a toothpick between the cloth and the button. If it's a four-hole button, you can either make parallel stitches or an X-style. Check the other buttons to see what matches. Make four to six stitches of either kind.

Wrap it. When you're done stitching, come up from behind the button once more without going through the holes in the button. Then loop the thread three times around the stitches between the button and the cloth. This makes a shank to keep 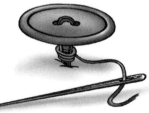 the button from floating all over the place. Run your needle and thread to the back of the fabric once more and knot it tightly there.

You're done. Sit back, admire your work, and resolve to shed those extra pounds.

Change a Tire

If you're reading this before you actually have a flat, congrats on your foresight. We have a little task for you to perform. If your car came equipped with a little L-shaped tire iron, go get it. Now fling it as far as you possibly can, preferably toward a large lake.

"I call those things punishment handles," says Pat Lazzaro, a certified mechanic and team manager of the Derhaag Motorsport Trans Am series racing team in Minneapolis. "They're good for teaching you a colorful new vocabulary, and that's about it."

Head on down to a discount store and look for an X-shaped tire iron (also called star wrenches). Check your owner's manual to see what size you need.

Spare Change

You won't be able to change a tire in 10 seconds flat—the time it takes Lazzaro's pit crew. "It's actually more difficult to change a passenger car tire than a racing tire," she explains. "With a street tire, you're usually dealing with pretty primitive equipment."

But that doesn't mean you can't change one like a pro. Here's what Lazzaro recommends.

Clear out of traffic. Get off the road as far as you can. If you can't immediately find a safe spot, drive very slowly on the flat until you can. A ruined tire is better than a dead you. Make sure your four-way warning lights are flashing.

Set the parking brake. This locks the rear tires. If it's an automatic transmission, put the car in Park. If it's a manual, put it in first or second gear. Dig out your owner's manual and check to see where to position the jack. If you're changing a rear tire, place a chock—a block or wedge to keep the wheel from moving—in front of the tire that's diagonally opposite to the one you're working on. That tire takes the brunt of the weight when you start jacking, and on a rear-wheel drive car, there's nothing braking it. If you don't have chocks, find a big rock and set it firmly in front of the tire.

Get your gear out. Remove the jack, lug wrench, and spare from your trunk. Pry off the hub cap with the flat end on your tire iron and keep it close—it's a good place to set the lug nuts so you don't lose them.

Loosen each lug nut by one full turn, no more. If the nuts are rusty, Lazzaro suggests giving them a shot of WD-40 or some other penetrating oil.

Otherwise, don't be afraid to drop a booted foot down on the end of the tire iron to get it started.

Know Jack. Position the jack according to the owner's manual and lift the car until the flat tire is still touching the ground a bit. If you lift it right off the ground at this point, the wheel may spin as you try to remove the lug nuts.

"While that's fun, it doesn't do much for getting the wheel off," says Lazzaro. Remove the lug nuts completely. Finish jacking the car up until the tire is just off the ground. Never jack the car up any more. The higher you jack it, the more unstable it is.

Ditch the flat. Take off the old tire. Position the spare on the lug bolts. Hand-tighten all the lug nuts. Lower the car until the tire just touches the ground, again to keep it from spinning as you tighten. Tighten one lug nut as hard as you can crank with the tire iron, then do the one diagonally across. This makes sure the tire is flush and won't wobble. Do the same with the remaining nuts. Lower the car completely. You're done.

One final note: If you're using a temporary spare (also called a donut), don't exceed the maximum speed stamped on the side, and get it replaced as soon as possible. They're only designed to get you a minimum distance until you can get the normal tire repaired.

Change the Oil

Besides being a certified mechanic and spokesperson for Bridgestone/Firestone's consumer education program, Pat Lazzaro is the first woman to complete the famed Jim Russell race car mechanic training program.

Plus, she's a former driver on the Dodge Shelby pro tour. Now she's trackside, working as the team manager for Derhaag Motorsports in the Trans Am series. She knows a thing or two about changing oil—one of Derhaag Motorsports' race cars takes 12 quarts of oil. "And we change it about every 200 miles," she says.

Thankfully, you don't have to do it anywhere near as often as Lazzaro's pit crew. But learning to do it yourself will save you big bucks. "Over time, it's a big cost-savings to do it yourself," Lazzaro says. And you'll be far from alone—one poll showed that 32 percent of Americans change their own oil.

There's one serious responsibility that comes with changing your own oil. It's called recycling. And it's important.

The Environmental Protection Agency estimates that 200 million gallons of used motor oil have been improperly disposed of in the United States alone. If that's not shocking enough, consider that just 1 gallon of used oil has the potential to contaminate up to 1 million gallons of drinking water. Check with a local garage, lube shop, or car dealership to see who takes used oil. Often you can even recycle the old filter.

Getting Ready

Before you begin, you'll need a few tools and parts. Here's the list: a small to medium adjustable wrench, an oil filter wrench, a new filter, an empty container that will hold at least five quarts (you can get a special oil-changing container with a cap at an auto-supply store), a funnel, a rag, enough new oil (check your owner's manual), and jack stands.

An important note: Sometimes you don't need jack stands to reach the oil plug and filter. You can reach them on certain models by lying in front of the car and reaching underneath. But if you do need to get under the car, *never* use a regular tire jack. You want to save a few dollars by changing the oil yourself, but not at the cost of your life. Regular jacks can slip and drop the car on you, Lazzaro warns.

Do It Yourself

Once you have your gear, Lazzaro offers this step-by-step game plan to use it.

Make the grade. Motor oils are labeled by grade. One common grade is 10W30, a general purpose, multigrade oil. That means it's good across most seasons and in normal driving conditions. The number before the W measures viscosity (resistance to flow) at lower temperatures, and the second number measures viscosity at higher temperatures. So, a 5W30 would work better at lower *and* higher temperatures than a 10W40. The higher the number, the thicker the oil. If you're unsure what you need, go by the owner's manual recommendations.

Go for the fake. Then there's the synthetic oil versus regular oil decision. In this case, fake is better than real. "Synthetic oil bears up so much better under adverse conditions," says Lazzaro. But, it's three to four times more expensive. If you drive in extreme temperatures—hot or cold—consider synthetic. Likewise, if you run your vehicle under heavy loads, like towing a trailer or carting your unemployed brother-in-law around, synthetic would serve you well.

Run the engine for about three minutes. Warm oil drains more easily than cold. Don't run the engine any longer, or you'll have to deal with searing hot oil.

Prepare the platform. Drive your car up on the jack stands if you need them. In either case, set the parking brake and put the car in gear or Park. If you have wheel blocks, use them. You don't want the car rolling around when you're under it or in front of it.

Drain the old oil. Place your shallow collecting container underneath the oil plug. The plug is hexagonal and sits on the bottom of the engine block on the oil pan. Unscrew the plug counterclockwise with your adjustable wrench. Oil is heavy and it'll come pouring out quickly, so keep your kisser clear. When the oil has drained, screw the plug firmly back in, but not so tightly that you strip the threads.

Remove the filter. Place the oil filter wrench around the oil filter. Turn it counterclockwise to remove. If the filter has been on for a while, it may be stuck. If, after all your cranking, it won't budge, you can drive a long screwdriver through the filter and use that to give you more torque in unscrewing it. Make sure you pierce the filter toward the bottom, well away from where it connects to the engine. There's a threaded post that sticks into the filter from the engine block, and if you hit that, you'll never get another filter on it again.

Put on a new one. Take a rag and wipe off the area on the engine around where the filter connects. It needs to be clean for a good seal. Dip your fingertip in some new oil and run it over the circular edge of the new filter. This keeps the filter from sticking when you go to change it again. Hand-tighten the new filter in place. Once you do that, turn it one-quarter turn with the filter wrench. Be careful not to overtighten or you'll strip the threading.

Fill 'er up. Pour new oil into the engine until the dipstick reads full. Start your engine and check around the plug and filter for any

leaks. Turn the car off and check the dipstick again. The oil level will have dropped some because the filter doesn't fill up until you run the engine. Add some more oil to top it off.

Ch-Ch-Ch-Changes

The engine on the Pontiac Bonneville had seized tighter than Scrooge McDuck's grip on a dollar bill when its owner brought it to Salem Boys Auto in Tempe, Arizona. After buying the car new, the owner had driven it 22,148 miles without ever cracking the hood to change the oil or check anything, says Mark Salem, owner of Salem Boys Auto and an ASE certified master technician.

Not to belabor the point, but 22,000 miles is *way* too long to go without an oil change. On the other end of the spectrum, many people change their oil too often, wasting money. The range between oil changes should fall between 3,000 and 7,500 miles, depending on how you drive, Salem says.

If you drive under 15 miles at a stretch most of the time, you should change your oil every 3,000 miles. If you split your driving time between city and highway and if your dipstick and oil cap show no signs of sludge buildup, you can stretch your oil changes to 5,000 miles. Just make sure you don't let it slide beyond that point.

Ninety-five percent of drivers fall into the 3,000 to 5,000 mile range, says Salem. The other 5 percent can go up to 7,500 miles. These are the people who are on the highway constantly—the traveling salesmen type.

One caveat: If you go over 3,000 miles, keep a sharp eye on the dipstick, says Salem. Most cars are a quart low at 3,000 miles. You can do real damage to your engine if you don't keep the oil topped off. Make a habit of checking it at each fuel filling.

Build and Maintain a Fire

In movies and magazines it always looks so perfect: A man and a woman cozied up on plush pillows in a darkened room illuminated by a toasty fire. The picture whispers romance. It sighs seduction. In real life, however, it can be a different story. A guy who doesn't know fire-building basics may be unable to get a blaze started, or he may initially succeed, only to have it quickly peter out—along with the romantic mood he was trying to create.

Bruce Springsteen once said that you can't start a fire without a spark. But the truth is, you need more than just a spark. The Boss probably just couldn't think of anything that rhymes with "kindling." So here's a handy checklist.

Tinder. Whether it's the sports section or the classifieds, newspaper acts as the tinder that gets a fire started. A lot of people wad it into balls, but a better method is to roll up single sheets of newspaper and twist them so they have a feathery end, says Ashley Eldridge, director of education at the Chimney Safety Institute of America in Ashland, Virginia. This creates a greater ability for air and flames to circulate around both sides of the paper, he says.

Don't use newspaper with lots of color or glossy newspaper advertisements in your fireplace, Eldridge cautions. Some contain heavy metals that can be toxic when burned.

Kindling. Twigs and branches or small pieces of wood sold by lumber yards typically are used as kindling. An excellent alternative is to place pinecones in paper bags, Eldridge says. They act as both tinder and kindling when lit, igniting a hot, fast fire, he says.

Firewood. Hardwoods such as oak, hickory, and locust burn longest because they are so dense, Eldridge says. Soft woods such as maple, fir, and spruce are also acceptable, especially in the spring and fall when the weather is mild and you're less inclined to need a fire that burns a long time, he says.

Regardless of the type of wood you burn, it should be seasoned enough that it is quite dry, Eldridge says. As fresh wood begins to dry, it gets check marks on the cut ends of the wood and cracks emanate from the center. The best time to buy wood is in the spring, which gives it plenty of time to dry out because you probably won't be burning it until fall or winter. If the wood is too fresh or damp, the fire uses a good deal of its energy to drive off moisture, creating less heat. And don't use treated wood, which can release dangerous chemicals when burned.

If you must store wood outside, place it on a pallet, not on the ground, advises Eldridge. Then cover it with a sheet of plastic.

Incidentally, those fabricated logs you can buy at the supermarket and elsewhere work fine, Eldridge says. "You have to be careful not to poke or prod them while they're burning," he

The Perfect Fire

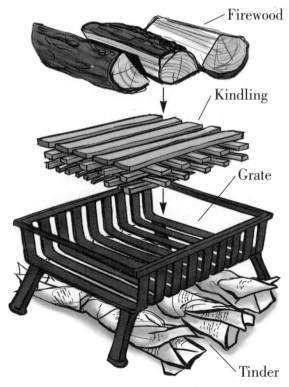

Firewood

Kindling

Grate

Tinder

cautions. "In some cases, they contain a binder that can be somewhat explosive. If you're one of these people who likes to fiddle with a fire, don't use them. But if you're someone who likes to just light the package and leave it alone, it's perfect."

Building the Fire

The first thing you should do when making a fire in a fireplace is to be sure that the damper is open, says Eldridge. The damper controls the flue—the vertical column in the chimney that contains the exhaust of the fire. Typically, there is a lever or chain in the damper. Forget to open it, and your house will fill with smoke.

If there is ash on the floor of your fireplace from the last fire, leave some of it for your next effort. "About an inch of ash under the grate is ideal," Eldridge says. As embers settle, they nestle into the ash and retain heat there.

Now it's time to build the perfect fire. Here's how.

Start spreading the news. Arrange at least three or four of those strips of newspaper you've twisted up under the grate, with the feathered tips facing the front. By the way, the grate should be no more than two-thirds the size of the fireplace, Eldridge says.

Play Lincoln Logs. Stack the kindling in opposite directions, log cabin–style. The bars of the grate typically run from front to back, so you would place your first batch of small kindling so that it is perpendicular to the bars of the grate, Eldridge says. "It's all incremental, done in successive sizes," Eldridge says. "The idea is to have sufficient kindling to cause the next larger wood to ignite."

After building up the first batch of kindling a couple of inches, add bigger sticks and branches of one to two inches in diameter and place them in the opposite direction across the smaller kindling. Your largest sticks and branches

Keeping Your Fire in Its Place

Here are some safety tips from the Chimney Safety Institute of America (CSIA) to help ensure that your firewood—not your home—goes up in smoke.

- Never use lighter fluid, gasoline, or any other flammable fuels to get a fire started. They are too combustible.
- Don't ever leave a blazing fire unattended. An errant ember is all it takes to start a fire.
- If you use your fireplace often, have a CSIA-certified chimney sweep inspect it every year. Spring is a good time to do so. Soot and creosote—unspent fuel that collects in a cool chimney flue—accumulate in a chimney and, if not cleaned out, can lead to a chimney fire.

come next and should be no more than four inches in diameter. Again, place them in the opposite direction across the previous layer of sticks.

Log on. Place a couple of small logs atop the heap. Don't start off with a big log, which could overwhelm your fledgling fire and snuff it out, Eldridge says. Nor should you use too many logs of any size all at once. "Even relatively dry wood will have 15 to 25 percent moisture," Eldridge says. Some of those logs will suck up energy and warmth from the fire as it tries to drive off that moisture.

Light your fire. Long matches and lighters will do the job, but Eldridge prefers lighting a rolled-up strip of newspaper. Then he presses it through the opening in the damper. By watching the smoke come off the paper, you can tell if it will go up the chimney or into your room. This method also creates an updraft that helps disperse smoke more quickly, he says.

After holding the burning paper in the damper a moment, light the newspapers you've placed under the grate with it, and your fire is under way, Eldridge says. Later, when you are confident that your fire is roaring along nicely, you might add a larger log.

Barbecue like a Pro

Nothing so embodies modern man in all his suburban sanguineness as the backyard barbecue. There, he can coolly demonstrate his prowess over a hot fire, wielding tongs and knives like a samurai warrior. He is master of the marinade, king of the grill.

That connection to food and fire may date back to caveman days when a guy ambled outside to kill his dinner, dragged it back, and threw it on a fire, says George Hirsch, chef, author of four cookbooks, including *Know Your Fire*, and host of a public television series by the same name. "I think that it has carried over since then."

Indeed, there are 2.9 *billion* barbecues every year in America, says Donna Myers, a spokesperson for the Barbecue Industry Association and editor of *The Backyard Barbequer*. Some 84 percent of families own at least one grill, she adds.

Tools of the Grill Master

You can buy charcoal, gas, or electric grills, but the first two are more common and effective, Hirsch says. Gas traditionally has been viewed as faster and more convenient. The trade-off has been that gas grilling produced less flavor. Charcoal was perceived as cumbersome, but more tasty. Those distinctions are blurring, however.

But the grill is only the beginning. A man needs tools to work with the grill of his choice. These include:

Tongs. Get tongs with long handles so that you singe the food you're cooking, and not your finger hairs, Hirsch advises. Tongs allow you to turn over meat or remove it from the grill without jabbing a hole in it, which lets flavorful juices escape, he says.

Spatulas. They serve the same purpose as tongs and are especially useful for moving fish or other foods that can fall apart easily, Myers says.

Basting brushes. These are used for dabbing on marinades and sauces. Hirsch recommends buying inexpensive ones and replacing them regularly.

Heat resistant gloves or towels. They can protect your hands from getting scorched, Hirsch says. He prefers a towel, finding it less cumbersome than gloves.

Instant-read thermometer. You stick this in the meat to get a temperature reading, then instantly remove it. Doing so enables you to avoid cutting into the meat to see if it is cooked all the way through. Good food safety practices dictate that a thermometer should be used with *all* meat to ensure it is properly cooked. Don't bother using a thermometer in fish, Myers says. Instead, stick a fork into the center and see how much it flakes. The flesh

Stacking the Odds

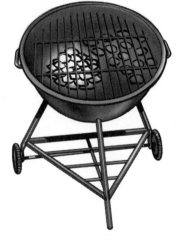

You can keep one section of charcoal cooler by spreading out the coals (shown on right). Conversely, coals should be bunched higher and tighter in another section to generate the most heat (shown on left).

should be opaque, not translucent, she says.

Grill topper. Many grills have grates that allow smaller foods such as vegetables and shellfish to fall below. A grill topper consists of a stick-resistant metal or porcelain plate with small holes. It is placed directly over the grid on a grill.

Charcoal Grills

This is the American classic. And like any true classic, it never goes out of style. Here's how to barbecue like it's 1959.

Build a briquette house. How many charcoal briquettes you use depends on how much meat you're cooking, but 25 to 30—about 2½ pounds—is a good rule of thumb, Myers says. It generally takes about 20 minutes for them to become sufficiently hot to begin cooking. Coals should be ashy gray.

If you are cooking for a long time, add 8 to 10 new briquettes to the edges every 45 minutes, Myers suggests.

Forgo the fluid. The use of lighter fluid is waning, and one reason is the increasing popularity of chimney lighters, Hirsch says. You place the cylinder-shaped device in the bottom of the grill, fill it with charcoal, place a piece of newspaper on the bottom, and light it.

When the coals have turned ash gray or white about 15 minutes later, empty them into the bottom of the grill and start cooking, Hirsch says. Just make sure to use a towel or to wear protective gloves when handling the hot chimney lighter, he adds.

Forgoing lighter fluid is more ecologically friendly and will result in tastier dishes, Hirsch says. Lighter fluid—whether applied

Wood You Believe?

Want to give your barbecue a little extra zing? Experiment with aromatic smoking wood chips. With a charcoal grill, mix the chips in with the briquettes, says Donna Myers, spokesperson for the Barbecue Industry Association. If your gas grill has a smoker box, place the chips there. Otherwise, place them in aluminum foil and set them in the ceramic briquettes at the bottom of the grill. Soaking the wood for 30 minutes in water before adding it to the grill will ensure smoldering and intensify the smoke flavor. Here are some of the woods to choose from and what they go best with, according to Myers.

Hickory: Ribs, burgers, and "anything that's not too delicate."

Mesquite: The strongest flavor, good with beef, lamb, and pork.

Alder: Chicken, lamb, game birds, fish, and pork.

Apple: Turkey, chicken, pork chops, sausages, and ham.

Cherry: Beef, pork, lamb, ribs, and turkey.

Maple: Ham, vegetables, pork, poultry, and fish.

directly or already added in presoaked briquettes—flavors your food to some extent, he says.

Book an indirect flight to taste. Much of your cooking should be done with indirect heat, Hirsch says. The idea is to leave some coals burning more slowly than others.

If you are cooking several foods at once, move those that are cooking faster to the slower-burning coals so they don't get dried out or burned. This technique is especially useful when you're cooking meats that drip a lot of grease, causing flames to flare up, Hirsch says.

Gas Grills

It even sounds manly: a gas-*powered* grill. Here's how to make your next barbecue a real gas.

Use ceramic briquettes. Most gas grills use either lava rocks or ceramic briquettes. Hirsch prefers the briquettes. Space them about an inch apart. Lava rocks are porous and absorb grease and drippings, he says. This permeates your food.

Go for the burn. Turn on the gas tank and all burners, then press the ignition, leaving the lid open while you do so, Hirsch says. Once it's lit, preheat the grill on high with the lid closed. In about 15 minutes, the ceramic briquettes should be hot enough for cooking. Most units contain a thermostat, but some are temperamental, Hirsch says.

Cool your jets. After you've preheated the grill, quickly sear (brown the surface of) the meat on each side, and then turn off one or more burners and cook your food over those burners, Myers says. There still will be sufficient heat to cook, but it won't be so intense as to burn or dry out your meal. This is especially effective for longer-cooking foods. During cooking, leave the lid up if you prefer a less smoky flavor, and down if the smoky taste is what you like, Hirsch advises.

Take some action on the side. Some gas grills come equipped with a side burner. They're worth the extra money, Hirsch says. "I have endless uses for it," he says. When you are cooking meat, for example, you can heat anything from a sauce to pasta on the burner.

Bits and Pieces

You're almost ready to show your neighbor who's the real king of the grill. Here are just a few more things you should know.

Grease the grill. Before you start cooking on a charcoal or gas grill, spray vegetable oil such as Pam cooking spray on the grill so that pieces of meat don't stick to it later. Do this when the grill is cool, Hirsch says.

Cook downwind. Try to barbecue downwind from family and friends, Myers suggests. "There can be quite a bit of smoke, obviously, when you're cooking," she says.

Marinate your meat. Studies suggest that grilling beef, pork, poultry, or fish can turn certain substances in the food into cancer-causing agents.

But in at least one study, marinating chicken for four hours prior to 20 to 40 minutes of grilling eliminated most traces of carcinogens. A good soak should work for beef, and it may work for pork and fish, too. Any marinade will do.

Go easy on the sauce. If you're using a barbecue sauce containing sugar—brown sugar, corn syrup, or molasses, for example—don't apply it to the meat until the last 10 minutes of cooking, Hirsch says. Otherwise, the sauce will get scorched.

Thaw all meat. Meat should be thawed in the refrigerator before cooking it on a grill, says Hirsch. If you are cooking a meat with bones, such as a whole chicken or ribs, thaw it in the fridge, then at room temperature for 20 minutes before placing it on the grill.

Treat your meat tenderly. Guys feel they have to be constantly poking and turning their meat, Hirsch says. Don't. This doesn't let it cook thoroughly.

"If you need to get your aggressions out, take a martial arts class," Hirsch says. Sear the meat and move it to lower heat. "You only need to turn it once."

Hone your skills. "Start simple," Hirsch advises barbecuing novices. "For example, if you really enjoy seafood but you're not that accustomed to cooking it, you might not want to start out by cooking a salmon fillet, which could break up if you don't have it at the right temperature.

"Start instead with something simple like a swordfish or tuna. Then gradually work your way up."

Sharpen a Knife

Call it the penknife paradox: The sharper a blade is, the safer it is.

You'd think a dull blade would be less likely to do any major damage, but the opposite is true. "A dull knife has a tendency to slip," explains Gary T. Randall, owner of Randall Made Knives, a knife manufacturer in Orlando, Florida.

On top of that, the duller a knife is, the more pressure you have to put on it to perform the task at hand. Toss in an unplanned slip in addition to the extra force, and "it can cut the hell out of you," Randall says. Look at it this way: A surgeon would never use a dull blade. Neither should you.

Choose Your Blade

The first thing you should determine, notes Randall, is whether your knife is even worth sharpening. If it has a scalloped edge, like a bread knife, you won't be able to sharpen it yourself without special hones. If you can't stand the idea of cutting your French stick with anything else, take it to a professional for sharpening.

There are also knives with serrated edges. You know, the kind that claim to never need sharpening. There's a reason for this claim—once they're dull, they're junk unless reground to factory specifications. Give these knives an honorable burial.

But, if yours is a good-quality blade, Randall suggests these tips to get your steel back in shape.

Get stoned. Buy two sharpening stones at your local hardware store. One should be a medium or coarse grit. The second needs to be a fine grit. The larger the stone, the better. Big stones cut down on the number of strokes you need to make.

Schedule a lube job. Put a few drops

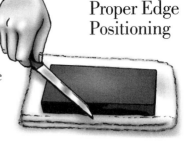

Proper Edge Positioning

of kerosene, machine oil, or mineral oil on the coarser stone. You'll hear some people griping about how you should never use lubricants because it plugs up the stone. Ignore them. Running a knife over a dry stone can burn the steel. "It's a good way to screw up a blade in a hurry," Randall says.

Stay put. Place the stone on a nonslip surface to keep it from moving around. If your tile countertop won't do the job, try putting a damp cloth between the stone and the surface of the counter.

Look sharp. Lay the knife flat on the stone at a 45-degree angle. Raise the blade so that it forms a shallow 20-degree angle to the surface of the stone. Sweep the edge from hilt to point along the stone, maintaining the same angle. It doesn't matter if you sweep toward or away from your body. Repeat until the edge is restored. Turn the blade over and repeat.

Clean it up. Use the fine-grit stone for the finishing touches. Increase the angle of the blade to 60 degrees and give it a couple of light swipes to remove any metal shavings still attached to the edges. Sharpen the blade according to your intended use. Gutting a fish, for example, requires a sharper edge. If it can cut a sheet of paper, the knife is good for cutting fish or animal flesh. Go easy if you're whittling wood. If the blade is too sharp, it won't hold an edge.

Practice. You're not going to get it perfect the first time. When Randall hires a new knife worker, it takes six weeks to bring that person up to speed on sharpening blades. And that's at a rate of 150 knives per week. "The practice is the real secret," says Randall, "but it's something every man should know how to do."

Get Rid of Pests

In *Annie Hall*, there's a scene where Diane Keaton telephones Woody Allen with an emergency at 3:00 A.M. When he arrives at her place, she asks him to kill a spider in her bathtub. He takes a look and concludes that the arachnid is "the size of a Buick."

"You got a broom or something?" he asks shakily. "A snow shovel?"

Instead, Allen grabs a tennis racquet and—flailing wildly—demolishes the spider and the bathroom.

Women expect men to stoically shoulder the burden of bashing bugs when they rear their ugly antennae. There are rewards. Keaton invited Allen into her bed after his heroics. There are, however, easier and less destructive ways to rid a home of pests. Or, for that matter, to get a woman into bed. But we'll save that for another chapter.

Battling Bugs

Bait them. Bait traps are effective and less toxic than sprays, pest control professionals say. Orkin exterminators use a slow-acting gel—also available over the counter—that the insect takes back to his colony to share with his pals, says Susan Kirkpatrick, director of public relations for Orkin Pest Control.

Whether you arm yourself with a spray or a bait, you need to be sure you have the right weapon for the right bug, says Stoy Hedges, manager of technical services at Terminix International and author of five books on various home-invading insects. Baits, for example, are useful in fighting many species of ants, but some, such as carpenter ants, aren't affected.

And neither a spray nor a bait will work if you don't use them near your quarry's home. Most insects prefer to hide in dark nooks and crannies. These often are located in areas between cupboards and the stove or refrigerator, under the fridge, and behind drawers and cabinets, Kirkpatrick says.

Shine a flashlight in these cracks and crevices to search for signs of your bug-eyed enemy, Hedges advises. Sometimes you can see their antennae poking out. In the case of German cockroaches, there may be black specks around the corners of a crevice. That's their feces. Regardless of what signs you find, this is where you must place your bait or aim your spray.

Drop acid. If you have roaches, use sticky traps to find out where they live and feed. Follow up by lightly dusting the roach highways and dens with boric acid, a widely available powder that kills roaches yet, if used correctly, is safe for household use. Apply it into cracks and crevices and around the motor of your refrigerator, which attracts the vile little critters because of the warmth. The roaches walk over the boric acid and then ingest it while cleaning themselves.

You can apply boric acid with a garden dust applicator, which is a small metal or plastic canister with a pump or a plunger usually found in garden supply stores, hardware stores, or mail-order catalogs. Wear a dust mask and goggles while applying boric acid. Do not swallow it, and don't get any in your eyes. Brush any powder that is visible after application into the cracks and crevices. Wash your hands afterward. Do not spread it in areas where small children or pets might ingest it. Avoid contamination of food and water. Carefully read all product labels for proper usage and safety precautions.

Suck 'em up. It may not be as satisfying as stomping, smashing, or poisoning your multi-legged tormentors, but vacuuming them sometimes works, and it's nontoxic. Be sure to throw the vacuum cleaner bag outside in a covered trash can. Vacuuming is especially useful against flying insects, which tend to land on windows where they are easy pickings, says Hedges.

Bug-Proofing 101

Of course, there is one way to avoid the unpleasant manly duty of bug squashing: Make your house inhospitable to the little pests. Here's how to do it.

Clean up. Insects generally like sweets, greasy food, and even beer, Kirkpatrick says. In other words, the same things as you. So wipe off the jar after you've poured honey, sponge off the table on which you spilled those french fries, and rinse out that beer bottle you're planning to recycle. Make it a point to sweep or vacuum regularly. Even if you're as fastidious as a maid in a four-star hotel, however, you may still have trouble. The typical roach can live up to 30 days off the glue on a postage stamp, Kirkpatrick says.

Store dried food in plastic or glass containers. Grain beetles and flour moths can be brought home from the grocery, Hedges says. By storing foods—especially pet foods and birdseed—in containers, any infestation can be limited to one food item.

Don't brown-bag. Cockroaches covet cracks and paper. Guess what? They get both in paper bags, Hedges says. Store bags in the garage or a closet outside the kitchen.

Don't be a drip. A colony of 200 roaches can easily survive on the drip, drip, drip of your leaky faucet, Hedges says. Repair any leaky faucets or drains.

Make a moat. If you leave pet food standing in dishes, place the dish in a bowl or saucer of soapy water to create a moat, suggests Hedges. This will keep roaches and other insects away.

Secure your trash. Keep lids secure on wastebaskets and garbage cans, advises Kirkpatrick.

The Critter Catcher

Catching a mouse in the house has you a little on edge? Then consider the job of Todd Hardwick. He operates Pesky Critters, a Miami business that, for a fee, will remove nuisance animals from your property. He snares alligators for free, re-releasing the little ones back into the wild and killing the large ones for meat and accessories.

Hardwick routinely receives calls regarding raccoons and opossums in garages and attics and armadillos on golf courses. But he also has removed "hundreds and hundreds" of alligators weighing up to 500 pounds from South Florida yards and swimming pools. "You're dealing with a cold-blooded, predatory reptile, and he has an attitude," Hardwick chuckles.

He also has pursued monkeys scampering across rooftops and trees and countless exotic escapees such as a 6-foot water monitor lizard that took refuge in a car engine compartment. One of his biggest challenges was extracting a 22-foot, 250-pound python from under a house. "That took two days of tunneling in under there and wrestling it into a sleeping bag," Hardwick recalls.

Hardwick has been bitten by some of the animals he's caught, but he has suffered no serious wounds. "I love my job," he says. "I'm saving people from animals and animals from people. I get to work outside under sunshine and palm trees all day, in or around the water. How could you ask for anything better?"

Caulk all cracks. Air-conditioning units, pipe openings into your home, and cracks and crannies in your cupboards and elsewhere are all places that should be caulked in order to block the immigration of insects into your home, Kirkpatrick explains.

Strip. Install snug-fitting weather strips on the bottom of exterior doors. Spiders, insects, and mice find that doors with poor-fitting weather strips provide them easy access into your home, says Hedges.

Check gutters. Make sure gutters are clean and that downspouts have splash guards or guards that move water away from your home so that puddles don't form near the foundation, Kirkpatrick suggests.

Keep your yard tidy. Keep mulch at least a foot away from your house foundation and no more than two inches thick, Hedges says. Eliminate piles of lumber and bricks. Store firewood away from the house. Keep tree and shrub limbs trimmed away from the roof and walls. Remove stumps and dead tree limbs, and fill in tree holes.

Do a screen screening. Check screens for rips, and be sure they fit well in windows, Kirkpatrick says.

But Do They Taste like Chicken?

Want to make the manly duty of killing bugs more palatable? Don't think of them as home invaders. Think of them as snacks.

In other parts of the world—especially in developing countries—people commonly eat bugs, says Donald Lewis, Ph.D., professor of entomology at Iowa State University in Ames. "They can be nutritious. How nutritious varies greatly with the insect."

Grasshoppers, for example, may contain up to 46 percent protein with a fat content of only 2 to 10 percent, says Dr. Lewis. Beef, by contrast, usually has a lot less protein and a lot more fat.

In the rare instances that insects are eaten in the United States, they are usually baked into a casserole or placed in cookies or breads. But if you're more adventurous, you can try frying, sautéing, or roasting them, says Dr. Lewis.

How to Catch a Mouse

Why dispatch a cute, furry little critter such as a mouse? Well, consider this: Being prolific breeders, one pair of mice in your home could potentially become hundreds of rodents if they have sufficient food and shelter. Their droppings can carry disease organisms. And, indiscriminate nibblers that they are, mice may even gnaw on electrical wiring and set your home ablaze, Hedges says. On the other hand, they also eat some of the insects you may be trying to eradicate. "We've caught them eating cockroaches off of sticky traps," Hedges says. Ultimately, you must decide if that's enough to offset their bad points.

Take them alive. If you have lots of mice, consider a multiple catch trap, Hedges says. Some hold 15 or more mice—alive. So if you don't like the thought of killing Mickey's cousins, you can always release your captives outside the house of the guy who races his car up and down the street.

In one variation of this type of trap, a mouse enters the device through holes on either side. When he steps on a trigger, a paddle slaps him into a holding chamber, Hedges says. No bait is necessary. "They investigate things that might potentially be a newer, better home," he explains.

Snap them up. This is the small, inexpensive trap with which everybody is familiar. You place some food in it, and when a mouse goes to eat it, he triggers a spring-loaded bar

Grasshoppers and grubs are particularly good candidates because they are easy to prepare and eat because of their large body mass, Dr. Lewis says. "A lot of small insects, such as flies, would supply little nutrition for the effort and be fairly unpalatable," he adds. Also, insects that are hairy or spiny should not be eaten. And although we can see where you might be tempted, you should never eat insects harvested from unsanitary sites, such as maggots from a sewer, cautions Dr. Lewis.

The strong cultural bias in North America against eating insects is likely to continue, Dr. Lewis believes. "Yet we consider lobsters a delicacy and we eat shrimp, and both are very close relatives of insects.

"When are consumers going to change their minds? Only when famine becomes widespread," he says. "I think it would take a catastrophic event to lead us to widespread consumption of insects."

you use to nab mice, you need to place it near their den. This is usually near food and water, such as in the kitchen. If you find their droppings—they often are in a corner—this is a good place to put your device, Hedges says. If you use a snap trap, put it so the trigger is facing or perpendicular to a wall, because mice usually travel on a path along walls. If you fail at first, move the traps around and try different baits. If you have lots of mice, use several different types of traps.

No Mice Allowed

If Mickey Mouse shows up at your door someday carrying a couple of large suitcases stuffed with cash he stole from his taskmasters at Disney, go ahead and let him in. But it's hard to imagine any other reason to let a little rodent into your house. Here's how to keep them out.

Seal the deal. Just as with insects, you need to seal all holes and cracks in your house, according to Hedges. "Every possible opening one-quarter inch or larger needs to be sealed. If you have a big hole around a water pipe, it's best to stuff some sort of wire mesh in there. Then use expanding foam to fill it in."

Guard your doors. Place tight-fitting weather strips on doors, including the garage door, which is a common point of entry for mice into homes, Hedges says.

Do a screen test. On foundation and attic vents, you need good window screens to keep out insects, but you also should add one-quarter-inch hardware cloth behind it to keep out mice, rats, and other small animals, Hedges says. Hardware cloth is a heavy-duty screen that can't be gnawed through by rodents.

Eliminate their habitat. Clean up yard

that slams down on him. About half of the mice who nibble on the bait escape death, but it's still relatively effective, Hedges says. For best results, use a trap with an expanded trigger—it's more likely to catch your mouse, he explains.

And what should you use as bait? "Cheese is the worst thing you can use," Hedges says. "Peanut butter and chocolate work well." So does malt-flavored hairball remover for cats. And since mice are always searching for nesting material, you can also tie a piece of cotton to the trigger with dental floss to ensnare your prey, Hedges says.

Go to a cathouse. If mice are a continued problem, consider getting a cat, Hedges says. They readily catch and eat mice.

Find their den. Regardless of what trap

debris and keep grass and weeds mowed, Hedges advises. If you have a mice problem and a lot of ground cover, such as ivy, consider replacing it with something mice can't hide in.

How to Catch a Bat

Drop any superstitions you have about bats being nothing more than evil little flying rodents sucking blood out of the unsuspecting on Halloween. Fact is, they're downright useful. A single bat can eat up to 2,000 annoying insects during his travels in one night. "Generally, they're good animals," says Harold Harlan, Ph.D., staff entomologist at the National Pest Control Association in Dunn Loring, Virginia. Still, even if you like bats, you probably don't want to be ducking as one flies in a panic around your house. Here's what to do.

Show him the door. Open a door or window and see if your visitor can find his way out of the house, Dr. Harlan suggests. If he's flying around rooms, he's searching for an exit. Contrary to popular belief, most bats see quite well, he says. But they rely principally on ultrasound to navigate and find food.

Wear gloves. A bat that is docile could simply be exhausted, or he may be sick—possibly with rabies, Dr. Harlan says. Don't touch the animal without wearing leather or canvas work gloves (this is true for all wild animals). If you are cleaning up bat or rodent feces, make sure to wear latex gloves and wet down the droppings before sweeping them up. This keeps the fecal dust down, which will help lessen the spread of airborne diseases like hantavirus, Dr. Harlan explains.

Scoop him up. If a bat in your house is not flying, use a broom or other object with a handle of at least two feet to try to scoop him into a coffee can or other container on which you can place a lid, Dr. Harlan says. Then take him outside and release him.

Kill, if you must. If you are bitten or scratched by a bat, capture him—dead or alive—and take him to your local public health office so it can be determined if the animal has rabies, Dr. Harlan says. Better still, if you can confine the bat to one room and close the door, ask the public health office to send somebody to you.

Banishing Bats

Once you get a bat out of your house, you'll want to prevent a return visit. First you must find out how he got into your house. Here are the three most likely points of entry, and what you can do to shut them down.

Attack the attic. If you have holes in your screens or other possible entry points for bats in your attic, repair them. A bat only needs an opening three-eighths to one-half of an inch wide to get in, Dr. Harlan says.

Some people put mothballs in their attics to drive bats out. It doesn't work particularly well, Dr. Harlan says. "If you put them right under where the bats are roosting, they will move to one side, but they may not move far," he says. If you insist on using mothballs or moth flakes, hang a fistful in a nylon stocking so you can retrieve those remnants that don't evaporate when you're finished, he says.

Cap the chimney. "If you have an open chimney, it's a good idea to have it capped with a screen that would exclude bats, birds, and other urban wildlife," Dr. Harlan says.

Check outside. Look outside for stained areas on the edges of eaves or under siding or shutters where bats may be roosting and gaining access to your home, Dr. Harlan says. All mammals, especially bats, emit a greasy, oily secretion from their skins. When the bats roost, you will see the discoloration and darkening on any porous surfaces they touch, Dr. Harlan explains. How do you tell if bats are hanging out on your eaves? Why, there'll be eaves dropping, of course.

Part Three

A Man of Style

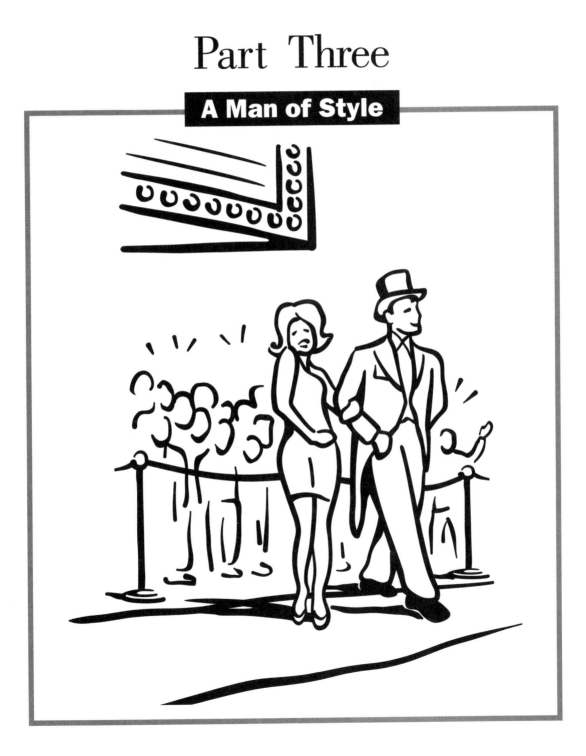

Travel Light

Nothing can spoil a trip like lugging luggage as heavy and cumbersome as a corpse. But that's not the only reason to travel light. Airlines have gotten pickier about the amount and size of both carry-on and checked luggage. And less luggage means shorter waits for baggage claim, less need for porters, and smoother Customs inspections.

The type of baggage you haul will go a long way toward either making your trip the equivalent of a boot camp drill or a walk on the mild side. Choose luggage that is lightweight, roomy, and easy to carry, yet durable enough to withstand punishment. Then it's a matter of packing smartly.

"You always need less than what you have with you," says B. J. Hansen, program director for the Adventure Travel Trade Association in Englewood, Colorado.

Here are tips from travel pros on how to lighten your load.

Plan ahead. Think ahead of time about what you'll be doing on your trip. Business engagements, any sports you'll be playing, the length of your stay, and how often you'll need to change clothes are things to consider, says James Ashurst, communications manager at the American Society of Travel Agents in Alexandria, Virginia. Doing so will better enable you to take clothing that you need and avoid packing articles you won't use and that would otherwise take up valuable space.

Be a weatherman. Similarly, by checking seasonal weather conditions for your destination, you can avoid packing items you won't use, says Hansen. If, for example, you're going to the Amazon basin, that flannel shirt you treasure won't be of use to you no matter when you visit.

Mimic Santa. Make a list—no need to check it twice—of things you plan to take on your trip, Ashurst says. This will make organizing your stuff easier, and the list will come in handy if your luggage is lost or stolen during your trip.

Pack suds for your duds. Either take laundry soap or buy some at your destination, says Hansen. By washing your clothes while you travel, you don't have to pack as many things because you need fewer changes of clothing. If there aren't laundry facilities where you're going, you can still clean some of your clothes in a hotel room sink or bathtub.

Protect your toiletries. Pack your toiletry kit in a carry-on piece of luggage rather than baggage you check, Ashurst advises. That way, if your checked-in bag is lost, you can still look presentable, which is especially important if your trip is business-related.

Buy when you arrive. If you neglect to take something you truly need, chances are you can find it at your destination.

"Let's say you're going someplace where there's a jungle and you live in Denver," says Tim Cahill, an editor-at-large for *Outside* magazine in Santa Fe, New Mexico, and author of several books, including *Pass the Butterworms: Remote Journeys Oddly Rendered.* "You're looking all over Denver for a machete. What are you doing? When you get to the jungle, you can buy a machete that's better and cheaper. I just see people worrying too much about what they take."

Packing It In

Once you know what you want to bring, the next hurdle is to pack it efficiently. Here's how to do it.

Start at the bottom. Pack your heaviest items, such as shoes and books, on the bottom of your luggage, suggests Hansen.

Pack tightly. Packing loosely wastes precious space, says Ashurst, and it causes your things to slide like deck chairs on a listing boat, wrinkling your clothes in the process.

Don't get in a jam. Pack your luggage

too full, and you may pop a zipper or a hinge, says Ashurst. "If you get to the point where you're standing on your suitcase to get the buckles closed, you've probably gone too far," he says.

Imagine your embarrassment when your briefs—the ones monogrammed with your initials and the slogan "Home of the Whopper" printed on the crotch—spill out onto the baggage claim conveyor belt.

Roll 'em, roll 'em, roll 'em. Roll pajamas, sweaters, and other casual wear into small spaces, where possible, Hansen suggests.

Have a color scheme. Choosing a wardrobe of basics will help you deal with space limitations, Hansen says. Pack clothes that will coordinate with one or two colors. "Jeans go with anything," Hansen adds.

Use every inch. Stuff your shoes with socks or underwear. You'll free up more room in your luggage and keep your shoes from getting squashed, Hansen says.

Take tiny toiletries. Pack miniature toiletries in small plastic bottles to save space and weight, Hansen suggests. Many pharmacies and supermarkets sell shampoos, colognes, and other such items in travel sizes.

You also can save those small bottles of shampoo and the like when they're included in your hotel room for use on future trips. Just be careful not to fill bottles to the top if you're flying because the pressure may cause the contents to expand and seep out. Pack them in a heavy plastic bag in case of leakage.

Leave room. Anticipate articles you might purchase at your destination—such as that machete—and take them into account when packing. If you're going to buy several

gifts or other items, include a second bag, such as a small duffel, that can fit inside your main luggage or be used as a carry-on piece, Ashurst says.

Packing for Adventure

Tim Cahill has traveled throughout the world, often under primitive conditions. Surely he's an expert on traveling light, right? "Everybody, including myself, packs too much. Then you have to lug that stuff all over hell," says Cahill, an editor-at-large for *Outside* **magazine.**

Here are a few things Cahill recommends that you do pack for an adventure travel trip.

Essential toiletries. **A couple of rolls of toilet paper, toothpaste and a toothbrush, an antidiarrhea medication, aspirin, antibiotic ointment, and moleskin for blisters.**

Fast-drying clothes. **You want clothing that dries quickly and wicks moisture away from your body. Wool and some synthetic materials work well, he says. Tencel is one of the synthetics that tends to be lightweight and fast-drying. "Try to stay away from cotton. It's going to get wet, and it never dries."**

A head lamp. **For camping or if you're traveling in a country with unstable electricity. "It leaves both hands free to do what you need to do at night," Cahill says.**

A small bottle of hot sauce. **"For bland or unappetizing food."**

A small short-wave radio. **Some aren't much bigger than a deck of cards, says Cahill, an admitted news junkie. In the event of a disturbance, "it's sometimes worth your life to find out precisely what is going on, such as where the demonstrations are taking place, and to avoid that area of the city," he says.**

Select and Open a Bottle of Wine

One of the surest marks of the urbane man is that he knows his way around a wine list. He confidently orders the right wine for the right occasion and artfully ministers over the arcane rituals that accompany the transaction, leaving women swooning and male business colleagues awed and impressed. It's like the old Spanish proverb says: "Water for oxen, wine for kings."

You don't need to be royalty, however, to master the basics of choosing the right wine. Keep a few simple pointers in mind, and you can pull this trick off with remarkable aplomb. And for many, it can become not only a hobby, but a passion.

"It's a lifetime quest between discovering new wines and enjoying different years and going back to the wines you like," says Camille Elroz, founder and president of the Wine College of America, a Chicago group that offers information and wine courses.

There are four types of wines: red, white, rosé or blush, and champagne and sparkling wines. The first two are by far the biggest sellers and will be the focus of this chapter.

Here are some of the red wines that Jim Reilly, wine columnist for a group of newspapers in Syracuse, New York, recommends trying, depending upon your tastes.

- Cabernet Sauvignon is considered among the best in heavy or dry wines. A red Zinfandel makes an excellent all-purpose heavy red wine, good with everything from steak to spaghetti to pizza to hamburger.

- Among light or fruity wines, Merlot is very popular. A Beaujolais "is a light, fruity, easy-drinking wine," Reilly says.

Conventional wisdom says that red wine should be served at room temperature. "When people talk about room temperature, they're talking about room temperature in the 1400s or 1500s, which was about 60 degrees," Reilly says.

Most red wines are best served at a cool basement temperature, he says. Some of the lighter red wines—Beaujolais and Pinot Noir—do better with a little chill. Put them in the refrigerator for 20 to 30 minutes before serving, suggests Reilly.

Among the most versatile white wines are the Rieslings, Reilly says. Some are fruity and sweet. Others are dry. It's a wine you can serve to novices or to connoisseurs, he says.

Among other choices, here is what Reilly suggests.

- Chardonnay wines are very popular and serve as a good general-purpose wine. A Chardonnay from Australia differs from a California Chardonnay or those made in France. Reilly prefers the French variety, saying they are drier and more subtle.
- Sauvignon Blanc wines are excellent— lighter, drier, and less fruity than a Chardonnay, Reilly says.

White wines should be served chilled. Store them in the bottom of your refrigerator or in an ice bucket.

Wine and Dine

The rules have become relaxed concerning which wines should be served with what foods, so don't be overly concerned about this, Reilly says. There are a few general guidelines to keep in mind, though.

"The stronger the food, the stronger the

wine," Elroz says. "The lighter the food, the lighter the wine. You need to create a balance between the flavors to avoid any one overshadowing the other." His recommendations:

- With heavy meals such as those with red meat, duck, or venison, serve a red wine such as Sauvignon or Pinot Noir.
- With lighter meals such as nouvelle cuisine, try a lighter red wine such as a Merlot.
- With seafood prepared in a rich sauce, have a Chardonnay.
- With lighter seafood such as grilled fish or shellfish, try a Sauvignon Blanc.
- With spicy food or food prepared in a sweet sauce, serve one of the sweet Riesling wines.

Mastering the Ritual

Once you've ordered your wine, it's show time. The waiter or wine steward brings the bottle of wine to your table, and all eyes turn to you. Here's how to handle the ritual with style and grace.

Confirm your choice. First, he will show you the label. Read it to confirm that it's what you ordered.

Inspect the cork. Next, he will open the bottle and present you with the cork. Some folks smell it in order to determine whether the wine has spoiled. Don't bother, Reilly says. Instead, inspect the cork to make sure the end is wet. This means that the bottle was kept on its side, so the cork didn't dry out and air didn't get in and ruin the wine.

Swirl and sniff. The waiter will then pour you a bit of the wine so you can be sure it has not spoiled. Swirl it in the glass to stir up the ingredients and smell the wine. Do so care-

---

A Grand Opening

Opening a bottle of wine gracefully is one of the signature moves of the suave fellow. Here's how to make it your move, says the Wine College of America's Camille Elroz.

- **Start by removing the foil above the ridge on the neck of the bottle with a knife. Cut all the way around.**
- **Then grab the top part between the knife and your finger and pull it away.**
- **Insert the tip of the corkscrew slowly, and turn until the entire worm part has entered the cork.**
- **Pull the end of the corkscrew slowly and evenly upward, and the cork will come out of the bottle. If it begins to bend, grab the cork with your hand and wiggle—don't twist—it the rest of the way out of the bottle.**
- **Sometimes a cork will start crumbling into bits and pieces. Push the rest of the cork into the wine, then pour it through a strainer either directly into glasses or a carafe, suggests wine columnist Jim Reilly.**

---

fully, however. "I've seen people swirl it around and spill it on the person next to them," Elroz says. If the wine is spoiled, it will have an acidic smell like vinegar.

Take a sip. If the wine smells good, sip it. If it passes the taste test, inform your waiter or wine steward that it's acceptable. If the wine has a suspicious smell or taste, however, send it back and ask for another bottle, Reilly says. "You should never be afraid of suggesting that something doesn't taste right," he says.

Once you've decided on a wine and approved it, pour it to the half-full point or a little higher in your glasses. "You want people to be able to swirl the wine in their glasses without spilling it," Reilly says. "So don't fill it one-half inch from the rim."

Get Great Service

You can spend a lot of money on dinner in an elegant restaurant, only to have it ruined by a surly, inattentive serving staff that seems to regard you with more contempt than a cockroach adorning a baked potato. Or you might spoil the evening all by yourself by acting boorish and superior to those waiting on you.

"There are people working in this business who have no business working in it, and there are guests who go out who really shouldn't," says Paul Paz, a professional career waiter for 18 years and president of the Waiters Association in Tigard, Oregon. "Both certainly are in the minority."

There are things you can do to make sure that your dinner out is an experience to savor. And it starts before you get to the restaurant.

Make a reservation. By reserving a table, you ensure that you get one, and you avoid disappointment and embarrassment, Paz says. Reservations are especially helpful when there is a special occasion, such as a wedding party or the closing of a big business deal. "Depending on your event, the restaurant may have some extra features that they will offer," such as birthday cake or a special bottle of wine or champagne, Paz says.

If it's a popular spot in an urban area, figure on booking a week in advance, advises Eleanor Widmer, Ph.D., a restaurant reviewer for the San Diego *Reader* for more than two decades, a public radio and public television commentator, and author of *The New Smart Dining in San Diego and Tijuana.*

Be flexible. If you call for a reservation at the trendiest restaurant in town on the busiest night of the week, you may not be able to reserve a table exactly when you wish, Paz says. Be prepared to accept a less desirable time.

Fridays and Saturdays are busiest, especially from 7:00 to 9:00 P.M., Dr. Widmer says. Your best bet is Tuesday through Thursday. Consider dining shortly after the restaurant opens—say around 6:00 P.M. Forget about Monday—some restaurants are closed, and those that are open may be more inclined to serve leftovers from the weekend, Dr. Widmer cautions.

Be patient. If your reservation is at, say, 8:00 P.M. and your table isn't ready immediately, don't sweat it, Paz advises. Sometimes diners who have preceded you linger longer than expected. "That goes with the process of dining out," Paz says. "We can't just throw out those guests preceding you."

If your table isn't ready within 15 minutes of your reservation, though, consider leaving, Dr. Widmer suggests. You can complain to the manager, but chances are that this will get you nowhere, especially on a busy weekend, she says.

Give your waiter clues. If you and your fellow diners have perused the menu and decided what you want to order, don't continue to sit there with your menus open in front of you. Instead, stack them. "You're sending a message," Paz says. "If you're really in a hurry, take the stacked menus and place them on the edge of the table. I train people to look for those indicators."

Be specific. "A lot of times, guests just don't make enough of what I call customer noise," Paz says. If you like your steak cooked until it looks as black and crispy as a smoker's lungs, tell your waiter. If you'd rather eat monkey brains than taste even a dollop of mayonnaise on your sandwich, speak up. The more information you provide the person serving you, the more likely the meal will be to your liking.

Consider the specials. Some diners think a restaurant's daily specials are old dishes the chef is trying to get rid of, or discounted, inferior fare, Paz says. It does happen, but more often the specials are dishes about which the chef is particularly proud. "There is some feature item the chef has discovered, or he has created a new recipe, or there may be a new product on the market he wants to present to his customers," he says. So if you want to order a meal that's likely to be top-notch, try one of the specials.

Give your waiter a second chance. If there is a relatively minor problem with the service—say, you had to wait too long for a coffee refill—don't suffer silently, and don't seek out the manager, Paz says. If you bring the matter to your server's attention, odds are it will be promptly addressed.

But if your server has been repeatedly remiss—no water refills, no bread, no checking back with you after you've begun your meal—talking to the waiter may be useless, Dr. Widmer says. They're either oblivious or they don't care, she says. Then the manager is your only recourse.

Don't make threats. One way to annoy your server and jeopardize service is to make negative references to the tip. It's rude to say things such as, "If this doesn't go right, you're not going to get a tip," or to tell the server that forgetting to bring a spoon with your coffee is going to affect the gratuity. "It's just tacky," Paz says.

Separate yourself early. A lot of servers—but not Paz—get irritated when customers ask for separate checks. Some computerized systems don't allow splitting checks after the data has been entered. "Where guests can help themselves is if they announce this at the beginning of the meal," Paz says. "When servers know in advance that there are separate checks to deal with, it's much easier for them to take care of it."

Passing the Bar

Good service isn't reserved only for fancy restaurants. You should expect it in your favorite bar as well. That means a bartender who is quick with a smile, attentive to your drink needs, and a good listener, says Bill Bade, who for 30 years has served as owner and director of the Midwest Bartender's School in Omaha, Nebraska.

If you're a regular, he will remember what drink you usually order. He also will place a napkin under your beverage, and he won't carelessly slap your drink down on the bar, Bade says. Nor will he allow a crowded bar to slow his service much.

"If he's a good bartender, he'll run a 20- to 30-foot bar and keep up on everything," Bade says.

Here's how you can show your appreciation to a good bartender.

Tip him. If a bartender is giving good service, tip him at least 15 percent. Much of their income is derived from tips, Bade says.

If you're having more than one drink, tip when you leave rather than after each drink, says Dr. Eleanor Widmer, a restaurant reviewer for the San Diego *Reader* for more than two decades.

That still leaves the question of how to ensure your bartender's attention, since he won't know that you're a generous tipper until you leave the bar. Dr. Widmer suggests sliding a couple of dollars to him before you order your first drink and saying something like, "I want you to take care of me."

Be polite. Don't rattle your glass on the bar to get the bartender's attention, Bade says. If he's occupied at the opposite end of the bar, walk over and ask if you can get service at your end.

Tip in Every Situation

Debate his singing or acting all you like, but about this there can be no argument: Frank Sinatra was a tipper extraordinaire. In his book about the crooner, *The Way You Wear Your Hat*, author Bill Zehme relates the following story. A parking lot attendant brings Sinatra's car to him, and Sinatra asks him what his biggest tip ever was. The kid says a hundred bucks. Not to be outdone, Sinatra slips him two hundred, then asks who gave him the C-note. Replied the valet: "You did, sir, last week."

For those of us not blessed with Sinatra's bankroll or his savoir faire, however, who we should tip and how much can be as perplexing as deciphering the tax code.

These days, it seems like everyone who does anything for you has his palm out. "The basic guideline is if the person is a professional, then you do not tip," says Hilka Klinkenberg, managing director of Etiquette International, a New York City company that provides advice on international protocol, business etiquette, and entertaining, and author of *At Ease . . . Professionally*. "Or if the person is a salaried employee, you do not tip." Examples of people who provide services for which you do not tip include airline attendants and personal trainers, though you may want to give the latter something during the holiday season.

Among the people who ought to be tipped—either routinely or during the holidays—are those who provide somewhat invisible services such as vacuuming the halls of your apartment building or delivering the morning newspaper to your door. These people often are overlooked, Klinkenberg explains, as are hotel housekeepers and wine stewards.

Sometimes people feel obligated to leave a gratuity regardless of the service received, but they shouldn't, says John Schein, president and founder of Tippers International and author of *The Art of Tipping*. "If you don't feel like tipping, you don't have to," he says. It's merely a custom, and a good one, he believes. "We can't get along without service people. How else are you going to let people know the service they provided was satisfactory?"

Tips also make up the bulk of some service industry workers' incomes. Still, if you don't think a tip is merited, don't show your displeasure by leaving pennies, advises Klinkenberg. It just makes you look small, she says.

It's not enough to show your displeasure with bad service by stiffing the staff on the tip, Schein says. Your act of protest could be construed as mere forgetfulness or ignorance on your part. For that reason, you should find a person in authority and voice your complaint, he says. This ought to be done sooner rather than later, Klinkenberg adds. If the service is lousy during a meal, for example, don't wait until you have finished eating to voice your complaint. Act quickly, and you can still salvage the evening, she says.

It's important, however, not to use a small tip to punish someone for events beyond his control, Schein says. If your meal was cold or not cooked to your liking, that's the fault of the chef—not the person serving you.

One distinction: Tipping is done after a service is rendered to show your appreciation. Money paid in advance, such as to a maître d' to secure a good table, is not a tip but more akin to a bribe, Schein says. Klinkenberg is opposed to this practice and says it often doesn't buy the intended result, anyway.

It's not just how much you tip that tells others you're a suave kind of guy. It's *how* you tip. Here are some pointers.

Your Tip Sheet

Here are guidelines for whom to tip and how much, according to Hilka Klinkenberg, managing director of Etiquette International. Make a photocopy, fold it, and keep it in your wallet at all times.

- Airport curbside check-in: **$1 per bag; more if your bags are like concrete**
- Skycap or train porter: **$1 per bag; more if your bags are very heavy**
- Airport shuttle driver: **$1.50 to $2**
- Parking valet: **$1 or $2**

- Taxi driver: **15 to 20 percent, depending on the professionalism of the driver and the cleanliness of the taxi**
- Limousine driver: **10 to 20 percent**
- Hotel doorman: **$1 to $2 for hailing a taxi; $1 for carrying heavy luggage**

- Bellman: **$1 or $2 per bag; $5 to $10 if your luggage is especially heavy or large; $2 to $5 for special errands**
- Room service: **15 percent—$2 minimum—each time (you can give cash or write the amount of the tip on the bill)**
- Housekeeper: **$1 to $2 per person per night (if you begin your stay late in the week and extend it through the weekend staff changes, leave the tip daily in an envelope marked "Housekeeping"; otherwise, leave one tip at the end of your stay)**

- Coat check: **$1 per coat**
- Bathroom attendant: **$1; $2 for special service**
- Waiter or waitress: **15 to 20 percent**
- Wine steward: **$2 to $5 per bottle (if he brings you a special reserved bottle, tip 5 to 10 percent of the cost of the wine separate from the dinner check)**
- Musicians, including strolling players: **$1 for a solo artist per request; $2 to $3 for a small group; $5 for larger bands**
- Bartender: **15 percent**
- Barber or stylist: **15 percent**

Be discreet. "It's so tacky when people are flashy and showy about it," Klinkenberg says. Sinatra was generous but not ostentatious when he tipped. "He never showed off. He would never flash a bill," Zehme quotes one Sinatra pal as saying.

Know when to fold 'em. "Don't hold the bills open," Klinkenberg says. "Fold them in your hand and just say 'thank you.'" Sinatra usually had others in his entourage do the tipping. But if he handed a tip to somebody personally, he folded bills three times into small squares that could be subtly passed in a handshake, according to Zehme.

Leave the table. If you are entertaining guests at a restaurant, try to pay the bill away from the table, Klinkenberg suggests. "Let the captain or maître d' know beforehand that during coffee and dessert you will be coming to them to pay the bill. Ask if they could please have it ready. Then excuse yourself from the table, pay the bill, and relax over dessert and coffee and leave." This enables you to calculate the tip without fanfare, she says.

Host a Dinner Party

Butch Reynolds learned an essential rule for hosting a dinner party—the hard way.

In 1995, the 400-meter world record holder was headed for a quick walk, shortly before presiding over a gathering of friends at his house. As he walked out of his door, a woman and her husband drove up next to him. They were officials from the International Amateur Athletic Federation, there to collect a urine sample in what's known as the knock and pee program.

Reynolds's back teeth were far from floating at that point. So the duo followed him on his walk. Dope testing rules require that officials keep an athlete in their sight until he springs a leak. Still no dice. The couple sat through two hours of the dinner party before the track athlete finally had enough juice to squeeze. The man stood by Reynolds's side as he filled a cup. Needless to say, there was a damper put on the party.

The rule Reynolds learned? The guests attending your dinner party can make or break it. Reynolds didn't have a choice, but you probably do. "You want to invite people who will get along," says Amy Mills Tunnicliffe, director of the Proper Manner, a corporate etiquette and business skills consulting company in Hingham, Massachusetts.

It's a sentiment that Alex Trebek, host of the quiz show *Jeopardy!* echoes. Trebek has developed a reputation for hosting some of the best dinner parties in the entertainment industry at his Studio City, California, home.

"Entertaining is a very simple thing," he says. "You pick the right people. You get them talking. You give them some good booze." Choose people who will contribute to the overall atmosphere, suggests Trebek, and pretty soon it's the host who will get the credit.

Of those people, make sure at least one is a gregarious type who can speak comfortably to almost anybody. "That way, if somebody shows up and has this esoteric background, that person can draw him out, make him feel good, and perhaps discover some elements that will endear him to the rest of the group," says Trebek. "And above all, try to keep the guests at ease so that they can each make a contribution."

The Host with the Most

Yes, if you choose your guests well, most of a successful evening is already guaranteed. But you're still the host, and hosting is in the details. Here are a few things to keep in mind.

Man the door. If you're busy, it's tempting to delegate door duty to someone else. Resist that temptation like a freshman resists 8:00 A.M. classes. "You should always be the first face they see," says Tunnicliffe.

Be prepared. Everything that can possibly be done in advance should be. When your guests start to arrive, the last thing they want to see is you rushing around juggling plates. "They feel as if they're intruding, even though they've come at the right time," explains Tunnicliffe.

Set the scene. "First impressions are everything," says Tunnicliffe. What that means is that your place should be spotless. There should be a cleared closet for coats. And for Pete's sake, clean up the bathroom and put out fresh towels. Guests should be greeted with something delightful for each of their senses. They should smell something good cooking. "Anything burnt is bad," says Tunnicliffe. They should see neatness, maybe some fresh flowers, a fire. They should taste—put an hors d'oeuvre and a drink in their hands. They should hear. Have some soft music playing, maybe some cool jazz or some unobtrusive classical.

Make the introductions. Again, being a host means hosting. If anyone at your party doesn't know someone else, it's your job to introduce them. At the same time, throw out some conversation bait. Tell John how Joe also is a die-hard Yankees fan. Give them a common ground to work with.

Present to impress. Good presentation of the food is essential. You don't even have to cook everything yourself. Concentrate on the main dish and go take-out on the side dishes. "Don't put it out in the little tin dishes," warns Tunnicliffe. Same with all the food. Dig out, borrow, or rent some good dishes.

Seat the guests. You're at the head of the table. The guest of honor (boss, celebrity, anybody who owes you money) goes to your right. Split up spouses. "They get to see each other all the time anyway," says Tunnicliffe. Alternate the rest of the seats by gender, that is, a man then a woman.

Leave the dishes. After dinner is over, just move into the living room with some drinks, dessert, or coffee. "It's not the time to jump up and start loading the dishwasher," says Tunnicliffe. Better yet, hire some help. "For a pretty nominal fee, you can have somebody else clean up," she adds.

A Graceful Ending

You've spent the evening glibly chatting among your guests. You've steered the conversation to safer topics when the subject of how men and dogs should be neutered came up. Now, the evening has come to a successful end.

Thank your guests individually as they leave, says Tunnicliffe. Make sure they know how much you appreciated their presence. Do not make them feel obliged to invite you over to their place soon. And don't mention how much work you put into the evening, even if they comment on it. Make it appear effortless, as if their company

---

Spam—It's What's for Dinner

Want to really knock your boss's socks off at your next dinner party? Want to make friends and influence people?

Well, the folks at Hormel Foods have the answer for you. The makers of Spam have thoughtfully developed a Spam Party Pack. It has everything you need to give your party a distinctive Spam flavor. And, we're sure, aroma.

Among the items in the Spam pack are:

- Spam invitations (Probably the same size as a pink slip.)
- A Spam tablecloth (What, no fine linen?)
- Spam paper napkins (As if you won't be wiping your face on the tablecloth.)
- Spam plastic ware (Stands up even to a rack of Spam.)
- Spam paper plates (Soft and safe for the inevitable food fight.)
- Spam balloons (Tie them to the mailbox at your neighbor's house the next time they throw a birthday party for their little brat.)
- Spam plastic serving tray (So you don't have to break out your good china.)
- And, just for you, a Spam apron (Sure to get you into the finer schools of cooking.)

We can have a few chuckles over the pungent pink pork product, but it's the people at Hormel who are having the last laugh. They've produced over 5 billion cans of the stuff since 1937, with 3.6 more cans added every second.

---

was the true success, not the amount of time you spent toiling over the meal.

Then slowly close the door behind them. Put your feet up and savor your accomplishment with a nice, cold beer.

Host the Ultimate Super Bowl Bash

Granted, most Super Bowl games hold as much suspense as an election in Cuba. But don't let this throw you if you're hosting a Super Bowl party. For some of your guests, the game is secondary to the socializing, eating, and drinking. So even if the game isn't memorable, your party can be—as long as you don't fumble the planning. In fact, it may be the one thing that keeps the day from being a colossal bore. Here's what you need to know in order to score points with your guests.

Covering the Spread

Perhaps more important than what you serve is making sure that you don't run out of food when you host a Super Bowl bash. It's one way to ensure that guests don't head for the exits if the game is a rout.

"You don't want to blow your food right at the beginning," says Martha K. Bindeman, owner of Finishing Touches, a party planning company in Bethesda, Maryland. "Once the whole food process is over, guests will leave." The trick is to serve munchies during the first half to quell folks' appetites a bit, then bring on the buffet at halftime, she says.

If you sent invitations to guests, expect to provide all the food and drinks yourself, Bindeman says. If it's an informal gathering of friends where everybody brings something, keep a list to avoid duplication. The host usually provides the main dish, but may opt to spring for beverages and paper goods instead.

If you're preparing the food yourself, strive for dishes that can be made in advance and easily reheated in the microwave so that you can mingle with guests, Bindeman says. "You don't want to be cooking anything when your guests are there." It also should be food that is easily eaten while watching television. Some suggestions:

- Chili is a great Super Bowl dish that can be prepared the night before the party, Bindeman says. When the game begins, simmer it slowly and enjoy the aromas that fill your house and whet your guests' appetites.
- Try fajitas. Put the fixings out and let your guests make their own, Bindeman says.
- Create a potato bar. "You just bake a lot of potatoes and don't put any toppings on them," Bindeman says. "You serve the toppings separately." Some of the choices you might give your guests: salsa, low-fat cheeses, caviar, and minced onions.
- Hye roller sandwiches. These are made with an Armenian soft bread, similar to a tortilla. Once again, guests can make their own from the ingredients you place out for them. These might include chicken, roast beef, salmon, lettuce, roasted peppers, and cheese, Bindeman says. The sandwiches also are sold premade by some grocery stores and can be rolled up and cut into two-inch morsels.
- A simple soup is good, especially if it's a cold day, which in most of the country it will be on Super Bowl Sunday. Bindeman suggests tomato or French onion without the cheeses. Serve the soup in mugs and eliminate the clutter of bowls and spoons, she adds.
- Old standbys such as deli cold cut platters and giant submarine sandwiches that can be cut into small sections are still popular at Super Bowl parties, says J. Schwartz, owner of The Entertainment Contractor in Los Angeles.

- Serve fresh fruit. "Even though at that time of year it's not the best, you can still do grapes and pineapples and berries," Bindeman says.
- A novelty football cake can be served for dessert. Brownies and cookies also are good, says Bindeman.
- Beer and wine are the unofficial beverages of Super Bowl parties, Bindeman says. Also have sodas and sparkling waters with limes for those people who don't drink alcohol. "Hot apple cider is a great favorite on a cold day with a lot of people around," Bindeman adds.

Schwartz agrees with the beer-and-wine observation, except if it's a particularly upscale group of guests. Then you might consider a full bar, he says.

Super Bowl Stats

Some Super Bowl trivia:

- **Americans reportedly eat eight million pounds of guacamole on Super Bowl Sunday, more than any other day of the year.**
- **Tickets for the first Super Bowl ranged from $6 to $12. Scalpers now ask as much as $5,000 for good seats.**
- **It's estimated that the median annual income of a Super Bowl ticket holder is $70,000, with one-third making more than $100,000.**
- **About 35 percent of those attending the game write it off as a corporate expense.**

Ready for the Football

Serving good food and drinks goes a long way toward making your party a success, but so does creating an appropriate atmosphere. "Little touches mean a lot," Bindeman says. "They just add to the festivity of watching the game." Here are some ways to do that.

Show your colors. Ask your guests to dress in the colors of the team they are rooting for, Bindeman says.

Decorate the joint. Display the teams' colors throughout your place the day of the game, suggests Bindeman. Or if all your guests are rooting for the same team, just feature that team's colors. Say, for example, the San Diego Chargers are one of the teams playing in the game. You might have napkins in the team's blue and yellow colors, or maybe balloons, she says.

Go for authenticity. Place the Super Bowl teams' pennants around the house or on the buffet table, Bindeman suggests.

Another option is to decorate with a few football jerseys and helmets, adds Schwartz. "You might even have a drawing where those items get raffled off at the end of the party."

Be a card. Scatter football cards around areas where food and drinks are being served, Bindeman says.

Let them eat cake. For dessert, serve a Super Bowl–themed cake in the shape of a gridiron, a football helmet, a football, or the like, Bindeman says. Only do the Cowboys cheerleader cake if it's a stag event.

Produce your own show. Instead of watching the lame halftime "spectacular" featuring some washed-up group lip-synching to the oldies, bring in your own entertainment. "Here in L.A., we have access to cheerleaders, like Lakers cheerleaders, who actually do a show," Schwartz says. Can't afford the Lakers Girls? Hire a strolling magician to perform during halftime, Schwartz suggests. Especially entertaining are those who can pick guests' pockets, he adds.

Play to a draw. Bring in a caricature artist to sketch guests during the break, Schwartz says. Since it's Super Sunday, he may draw them wearing football uniforms or something else consistent with the theme of the day.

Choose the Right Beer

Archaeology has provided us with some wonderful finds. King Tut's tomb. The remains of Pompeii. Lost cities of the Aztecs.

But the bone boys really got down to business when they found a 4,000-year-old Mesopotamian clay tablet covered with inscrutable writings. A great deal of scholarly effort was put forth to decipher the cryptic markings. After the translation was complete, they were undoubtedly pleased at their effort.

It was a recipe for beer.

Not just any old beer, either. It was a formula handed down from the god Enki himself. And it proves what any guy has always known in his heart—beer has always been an integral part of civilization.

Beer has also been a force in history on this side of the world. The Mayflower may not even have landed at Plymouth Rock if it was carrying more beer. An entry in the diary of a passenger aboard the famed Pilgrim vessel explains the unplanned landing. "We could not now take time for further search . . . our victuals being much spent, especially our beer . . ." it read.

Even much of the Declaration of Independence was created in the company of beer. Thomas Jefferson crafted a large part of the document in Philadelphia's Indian Queen Tavern. Jefferson also experimented with brewing techniques himself during his retirement at Monticello.

Know the Players

Fast-forward to today. Now is a great time to be a beer drinker. There are more than 1,300 breweries in the United States, says Matthew A. Hein, director of statistical and information services at the Beer Institute, the offi-cial trade association representing the major American brewers. This is the highest number of breweries since before the days of Prohibition. And the number is growing, with the explosion of microbreweries and brew pubs. In fact, in 1997, the United States surpassed Germany to become the country with the highest number of breweries in the world.

So, great. There's a whole bunch of high-quality beer available. But how do you distinguish between one and the other? A quick lesson in beer styles will help here.

Ales. Ah, the very word warms the cockles of our hearts. Ale is brewed through warm fermentation and is a top-fermenting brew, so called because the yeast floats to the top. Ales often have a much more complex flavor and a fruitier aroma because of the warm fermentation process. You'll also hear terms describing specific types of ale. Bitter is a British term for an ale made with a higher proportion of hops. India Pale Ale or, simply, Pale Ale is an ale originally made to withstand the journey to the Indian Empire. The higher alcohol content and hopped-up recipe meant the beer could suffer some degradation with traveling and still be drinkable.

Lagers. These are probably the ones you're most familiar with, as lagers make up the majority of the big labels. Lagers are brewed cold. The yeast stays at the bottom, so it's a bottom-fermenting beer. Lagers usually taste clean and clear with little aftertaste. Pilsner beer is a golden-colored lager. Bock beer is a deep, amber-colored lager. Bocks are generally considered an autumn or winter beer. In general, lagers, unless they're laced with preservatives, are best drunk soon after bottling. Unlike many other styles, they do not mature in the bottle. So, if anyone gives you a hard time about cracking open another one, simply arch an eyebrow and explain that the freshness clock is ticking on this particular beer.

Lambics. These are a group of very aromatic beers made from wild yeast rather than the typical cultured varieties. (It's kind of like the difference between John Belushi and Sir John Gielgud.) As a result, the taste of each beer is slightly different each time it's made. It also has at least 30 percent wheat in its mash, the rest being malted barley. Lambics are often the base of fruit beers, such as raspberry.

Porters and stouts. These are dark, dark beers, sometimes almost black. The malts in these beers are cooked to an almost burnt texture, giving the beer its distinctive flavor. Many people think that stouts and porters have a higher alcohol content because of the strong flavor. Not necessarily true. Although these beers often do have a more potent kick, some brands, such as Guinness, actually have relatively low alcohol contents. Porters and stouts are great beers to accompany spicy or strong-tasting foods. Their robust flavor stands up well to atomic chicken wings or liverwurst and onion sandwiches.

Wheat beers. In addition to the normal malted barley, wheat beers have a high proportion of—you guessed it—wheat. The result is a pleasant tartness (nothing wrong with pleasant tarts) that adds a unique taste and makes these beers very thirst-quenching. If you're traveling through Europe or deep within the import section of your local beer store, you may see these beers called weiss (German for "white") or weissbier (you figure it out).

Finding an Opening

Brett Stern is our kind of guy. He wrote a book called *99 Ways to Open a Beer Bottle without a Bottle Opener*. It should be required reading at every university. Here are five of his most creative suggestions.

Use the car door. Grab your beer, head out to the driveway, and open the car door. If it has a U-shaped latch plate, stick the cap under it and pry it open like you used to on those old Coke machines.

Bet the house. Unlock your house door and pop the cap in the slots of the door lock. Same action as above. Wave the open bottle at your neighbors and invite them over for one.

Select a golf iron. Any number will do, even the one your boss is currently using. Place the lip of the blade under the cap. Put your thumb on the cap. Pull up with the club and push down with your thumb.

Catch a brew. Grab your son's catcher's mask, ideally when he's not wearing it. Place the cap between two closely spaced wires in the frame. Pry off. This also works with a football helmet and a hockey mask.

Open it on the fly. This is a tough one; it's only for those in dire need. Undo your fly. Snug the metal tab under the lip of the cap. Use the glass bevel under the lip for leverage. With a sideways motion, pry the cap off. Try to remember to zip up afterward.

Choosing a Beer

Walking into a pub and saying, "Gimme a beer" is a lot like saying to an automobile salesman, "Gimme a car." Just because your father only kept bland, mass-produced, lawn-mowing beers around doesn't mean that's a tradition you need to continue.

But with new beers hitting the market almost every day, it can be tough to separate the wheat from the weak.

"I see men all the time standing with their eyes wide open with a wall of beer in front of them," says Christopher M. Bird, registrar of the Siebel Institute of Technology in Chicago, one of the world's leading schools of brewing. When you're in that situation, it's a perfect time to develop a sense of adventure, adds Bird, who also instructs at Siebel.

"That's the fun part," Bird says. "You really don't know what you're getting until you try it." Some stores even encourage your beer forays by allowing you to mix six-packs. Some also have six-packs already mixed for you.

You also may have a beer expert right in the store—the sales staff. Chances are very good that they sample their own wares, says Bird, and can fill you in on such matters as which beers are the freshest and which are their favorites. Avail yourself of their hard-earned knowledge.

Following are some other points that Bird recommends that you keep in mind.

Stay in the dark. Don't go to a store that stacks its beer in the window. Sunlight breaks down beer and can turn it skunky. You know if it's in the window, it'll get cycled back into the regular stock.

Have a glass eye. Metal cans impart their flavor to the beer. Glass is inert, and you taste just the product. This is not to say that cans don't have their uses. They're easier to take on outings because they're lighter. They cool faster (but they also warm faster). But if it's flavor you're after, buy bottles. But not just any bottles: Green ones let in more light than brown ones. Your best bet for fresh beer is going to come in a brown bottle.

Use the right glass. This time, we're talking about the glass you pour your beer into. It matters. The flavor and aroma of your beer can be affected depending on the shape of the glass you use. See the accompanying illustrations to match your favorite beer with the right glass.

Be systematic. Rather than haphazardly trying a beer here and a beer there, organize yourself. Arrange your purchases for, say, a month to all come from the same country. Or buy by the type of beer. Make January ale month, February porter month, March lambic

Home Is Where the Hops Are

It seems every guy has a horror story to tell about trying a buddy's first batch of home brew. For good reason. Until relatively recently, home brewing was, at best, an imperfect pastime.

"It used to be easy to make lousy beer," explains Mark Henry, owner of Evergreen Brewing Supplies in Bellevue, Washington, and author of *The Art of Brewing Beer.*

No longer. The selection and quality of home-brewing supplies and ingredients has never been better. What was once solely the realm of neo-hippies and homesteaders is now mainstream. "It's a popular hobby and a damn good one," adds Henry. "Beer is near and dear to most guys' hearts."

Plus, your buddy's eyes won't glaze over when you introduce him to this hobby instead of your stamp collection.

Here's what you'll need to get your first batch a-brewing: a high-quality hopped malt extract syrup such as

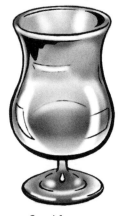

Tulip-Shaped

Good for:
Lambic
Belgian beer

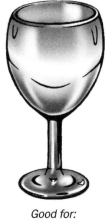

Goblet

Good for:
Porter
Stout

Coopers, yeast, an air lock with a bored rubber stopper, a siphoning tube, a 1½-gallon pot, a funnel, and a 5-gallon glass or plastic jug that your rubber stopper fits into. Toss in some empty bottles and a capping device, and you're loaded for beer.

The benefits of home brew include:

- **It's simple.** Beginner kits walk you through every step.
- **It's fast.** Four hours of actual work, and you're done. About a month later, you're drinking your first batch.
- **It has endless variety.** With 36 major styles of beer and 70 to 80 substyles, you can brew a long time and never repeat yourself.
- **It's cheap.** About $100 will set you up in fine style with all the gear you need. Choose the economic route by buying a kit that uses plastic instead of glass, for example, and it'll cost you about half that.

month, and so on. Or you can even make a trip around the world by buying a beer from a different country each time. Mark them off on your map as you complete your sudsy global trek.

Study hard. Many community colleges, large beer retailers, and brew schools offer taste testings where they will introduce you to samples of each type of beer. Hey, school was never so good. There are also tons of beer festivals popping up. At many of these festivals, brewers are on hand in person to explain to you the intricacies of their products. Tap into their brains as you tap into their kegs.

Take it on the road. When you're in a bar or pub, don't just order the first advertisement that comes to mind. "Nine times out of 10, people are drinking a marketing program instead of a beer," says Bird. Instead, find out what they have on tap. Choose one you haven't tried before, or ask the opinion of the bartender. You're almost assured he has spent some time under his spouts and can tell you the characteristics of each.

Pilsner

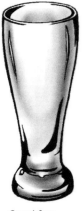

Good for:
Pilsner
Lager
Wheat beer

Traditional Pub Pint

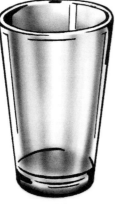

Good for:
Ale

A Rich Tradition

By spending some time learning more about beer, you are becoming part of a noble heritage of fellow beer-lovers. From ancient men to monks in the Middle Ages to the founding fathers of the United States, beer has been known and loved.

So loved, in fact, that at times men have been paid for their labor in beer. Hey, maybe some traditions should be revived.

"I don't know," says Bird. "I'm sure your wife wouldn't agree if you came home with a good buzz on instead of a paycheck."

Well, you don't know until you try, now do you?

Mix Drinks like a Bartender

There are some distinct advantages to throwing a bash at home rather than taking it out on the town. First, it's cheaper. But even better, you get to create your own environment, says Scott Young, creator of the Extreme Bartending Video Training Series and long-time bartender at one of Vancouver's hottest nightclubs, The Roxy.

The first thing you need to do is make sure you're stocked up, says Karl Kozel, a bartender at Manhattan's ultrachic Gotham Bar and Grill. We have some recipes for most of the timeless classics coming up. Make sure you have the booze and mixes to make them. Plus, get bottles of the most popular stand-alone liquors. Kozel suggests mainstays like vodka, a single-malt scotch, and bourbon or whiskey as bare necessities.

A couple of specialty items such as Amaretto, Triple Sec, and brandy are also nice. "You don't need big bottles of these because you're not going to use them that often," says Kozel. And make sure you have the gear to be an amateur mixologist. You can buy basic bartending kits, complete with shakers and jiggers, at many department stores and specialty shops, he says.

A Word to the Wise

No crash course in bartending would be complete without a mention of your duties as a responsible host. In some areas, the law holds you responsible for anything that happens to your guests if you get them plastered and they run into trouble on the way home. But no matter what the law says, "you're the host. It's your responsibility morally to look after your guests," states Young.

Here are some other things to keep in mind.

Set the tone. "Make people aware of what kind of party you want to have," suggests Young. If it's wild and crazy, so be it. If it's a more intellectual, sedate kind of evening, let Bluto and his buddies know.

Be creative. Young once won a bet for a raise with his boss that he could mix a drink in every possible color. He even got silver. Point is, you didn't get your chili recipe right until you experimented. Same with drinks. Don't be afraid to play with proportions a bit until you turn it into your signature mix.

Handle the goons. Some people just get way too rowdy after a bit of liquid courage. You're the host. You deal with it. "Do it in private," suggests Young. Take the lout aside, look him in the eye, and nicely tell him that what he's doing isn't cool. If that doesn't work, recruit his quieter friend to calm him down. "Tact and a little bit of discretion go a long way," he says.

The Ultimate Martini

Why does the martini crest the pinnacle of American mixology? Why did it become as much a legend as a drink? Because it speaks to the essence of American culture, says Lowell Edmunds, Ph.D., professor of classics at Rutgers University in New Brunswick, New Jersey, and author of *Martini, Straight Up: The Classic American Cocktail*. It is, as we are, classic yet individual. Sensitive yet tough. It separates us yet unites us. It is us, in a beautifully shaped glass.

Dr. Edmunds has been studying martinis since the 1970s, both academically and, on suitable occasions, empirically. So, after decades of thorough research, does he know how to make a truly great martini?

"Everybody claims that they make the best martini," says Dr. Edmunds. "Of course, I really do make the best." Here's his recipe.

Freeze your glass off. A martini glass should be kept in the freezer until you're ready to use it. Always have two—just in case.

Get some gin. Don't even think about vodka. Yes, it's the rage, but it isn't a real mar-

The Recipes

Here are recipes for five tried-and-true drinks that every at-home barkeep should know how to make, courtesy of Scott Young, creator of the Extreme Bartending Video Training Series.

Bloody Mary

1	*dash lemon juice*
2	*drops Tabasco*
1½	*ounces vodka*
2–3	*shakes of Worcestershire sauce*
3–4	*ounces tomato juice*

Shake the lemon juice, Tabasco, vodka, Worcestershire sauce, and tomato juice in a mixing glass filled with ice. Strain the mixture into an ice-filled highball glass. Add salt and pepper to taste. Garnish with a lemon slice.

Margarita

1	*dash lime juice*
4	*parts sour mix*
2	*parts tequila*
1	*part Triple Sec*

Blend together the lime juice, sour mix, tequila, and Triple Sec. Serve over ice in a margarita glass.

You can make this a frozen margarita by tossing the mixture in a blender with a handful of ice. Garnish with a lime slice.

Manhattan

1½	*ounces rye*
½	*ounce sweet vermouth*

Fill a mixing glass with ice. Pour in the rye and vermouth, stir, and strain into a chilled martini glass. Top with a cherry.

Tom Collins

1	*ounce gin*
3	*ounces lemon juice*
	soda water

Pour the gin and lemon juice into a Collins glass filled with ice. Top off with soda water. Garnish with a lime slice.

Whiskey Sour

½	*cup lemon juice*
2	*ounces rye*
½	*teaspoon sugar*

Fill a mixing glass with ice. Add the lemon juice, rye, and sugar. Shake, then strain into a sour glass filled with ice. Garnish with a slice of orange and a cherry.

---

tini. Edmunds uses Beefeater. Tanqueray is another good choice.

Verify your vermouth. Vermouth comes in red and white. You want white. Edmunds uses Noilly Prat or Martini and Rossi.

Go six to one. Six parts gin to one part vermouth, that is. Get a glass martini pitcher. Fill it with ice. Don't use metal—it picks up

odors and flavors. Let it sit for a minute until the pitcher is cold, then pour out the melted water (but leave the ice in). If you're making martinis for two, pour in six ounces of gin and one ounce of vermouth.

Banish Bond. "Shaken, not stirred," is how 007 orders his. He's fictional, you're not. Though experts debate this to tears, Dr. Edmunds quotes the theory of late U.S. historian and critic Bernard Devoto: "This perfect thing is made of gin and vermouth. They are self-reliant liquors, stable, of stout heart; we do not have to treat them as if they were plover's eggs." So, stir it gently. Let it sit for at least a minute to get supercold.

Pour and peel. Get your glasses out of the freezer and pour. Don't pour the ice from the pitcher; the drink is already cold and so is the glass. Peel about a three-quarters-inch piece of lemon rind and twist it over the drink until drops of lemon oil fall in. If you want to make it pretty, make a lemon zest. That's a curly, thin piece of peel that sits in the drink.

Add green olives. Dr. Edmunds puts his olives on the side, not in the drink. Either way, don't use the bottled ones from the supermarket. "Those are an abomination," says Dr. Edmunds. Go to an upscale deli and find some real ones. Niçoise, Green Lucque, and Picholine are all good va-

Tricks of the Trade

You say that you can pour a drink or two. So can a monkey. If you really want to distinguish yourself from the animal kingdom, take a few tips from Scott Young, creator of the Extreme Bartending Video Training Series.

Remember the movie *Cocktail* with Tom Cruise? That's extreme bartending—with a few Hollywood exaggerations and inaccuracies.

We asked Young for a few tricks to jazz up your time behind the bar.

The straw flip. Don't just plunk a straw in a drink—flip it in. Hold the straw between your thumb and index finger, about a quarter of the way down. Pitch it up in the air in front of you, letting it rotate once—or several times—before it lands in your other hand. Then place it in the drink.

The lime toss. Hold the drink in your left hand out in front of you and slightly to the left. With your right

Sour

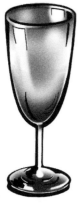

Good for:
Whiskey Sour
Apricot Sour
Amaretto Sour

Collins

Good for:
Tom Collins
John Collins
Red Death
  (or Red Devil)
Hot Toddy
Long Island Iced Tea

Rocks

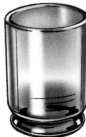

Good for:
B-52
Mudslide
Rusty Nail
Black Russian
Any liquor on the rocks,
  either by itself or with
  a splash of a mixer
(Also known as an old-
  fashioned glass.)

Margarita

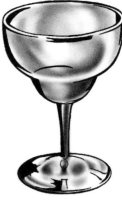

Good for:
Margarita
Daiquiri

hand, toss the lime behind your back and over your left shoulder. Catch it in the glass. Cushion the landing slightly, or you'll get wet. Practice with an empty glass.

The glass stack. This is a really impressive one. You need short, flat-bottomed glasses. The heavier the glass, the better. Fill three glasses with ice. Hold one glass in your left hand. Take a second and place it on the lip of the first one, just over halfway across the bottom glass. You might have to hunt a bit to find the balance point. Then take a third glass and balance it on top of the second one, a touch over halfway in the opposite direction. Once they're balanced, pour your booze and mix into each glass. Garnish and straw the drinks while you're still balancing them.

That should get you started. Just remember: "Anybody can mix drinks," says Young. "It's a waste of time if you're not doing something cool. Good luck and serve it with style."

rieties, although they might be very difficult to find.

Enjoy the experience. A martini is a sipper, not a shooter. "You have to take your time," says Dr. Edmunds. Sit back, sigh, toast your partner, and think good thoughts.

The Life of the Party

One final note—as bartender, you're also social director. "People expect you to do the entertaining," says Young. And all bartenders need a quick supply of good jokes. Here's one to get you started. After that, you're on your own.

Three vampires walk into a bar. "I'll have a pint of blood," says the first vampire. The second one says, "I, too, will have a pint of blood." The third one says, "I will have a pint of plasma."

"Okay, then," says the bartender. "Let me get this straight. That's two bloods and a blood light?"

Brandy Snifter

Good for:
Brandy
Cognac served
   straight up

Martini

Good for:
Martini
Manhattan served
   straight up
Cocktails such
   as Gibson,
   Gimlet, Bacardi
   Cocktail, and Kamikaze
(Also known as a cocktail glass.)

Highball

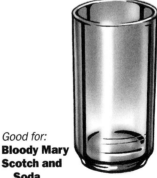

Good for:
Bloody Mary
Scotch and
   Soda
Rum and Coke
Screwdriver
Other basic drinks
(Also known as a
   straight glass.)

Make a Memorable Toast

Most guys probably don't give much thought to the subject of toasts—after all, how often do you have to make one? But knowing a bit about toasts now—when to offer one and how to do so correctly—can spare you grief later. "When it does come up, it panics you because you don't know what to do," says Debbie Horn, manager of education and club administration for Toastmasters International, an organization of clubs in more than four dozen countries whose members strive to improve their public speaking skills.

Occasions where you may be called upon to offer a toast include wedding receptions and anniversary and retirement parties. "Any time where you're gathering to honor or recognize someone, usually there's a toast involved," Horn says.

A toast normally bestows best wishes or hopes for health, happiness, or good fortune. "A toast can be serious, witty, sentimental, or even poetic," Horn says. "It depends on the person who prepares and gives it."

The Perfect Statement

So few toasts are memorable perhaps because people don't give much thought to what they will say, says Hilka Klinkenberg, managing director of Etiquette International, where she advises clients on such matters. So don't speak off-the-cuff.

Here are some other things to keep in mind.

Stand up. Unless you are in a small, informal group of eight or less, stand up when offering a toast, Klinkenberg advises. Doing so should enable you to command enough attention to quiet everybody down.

Get to the point. Keep it short and simple, says Klinkenberg. Limit your words to three sentences. If you are regaling guests with an anecdote about the recipient, that may not be possible. Even then, however, keep the toast to a minute or two, Horn suggests. The simplest words are perceived as the most sincere, Klinkenberg adds.

Strive for eloquence and wit. Don't turn your toast into a roast, advises Klinkenberg. It should be appropriate to the occasion, flattering, and even memorable, if possible.

Make it personal. "The nicest toasts are the ones that are personalized by the giver for the recipient or the occasion," Horn says. You can do this by including a personal story about the recipient or the occasion, or even by using an appropriate quotation.

Make eye contact. When offering the toast, make eye contact with the guests. As you are concluding your remarks, make eye contact with the recipient, Horn advises.

End on a positive note. A toast should be upbeat, Klinkenberg says. Lead the audience to a conclusion by clinking your glass to another or by asking guests to raise their glasses with you.

Rules to Speak By

Nothing will kill a festive occasion faster than a droning or inappropriate toast. Here are some ways to avoid common mistakes.

Wait your turn. No toasts should be made until the host has the opportunity to offer one. If it's clear he's not going to, discreetly ask his indulgence to offer a toast, Klinkenberg says.

Stay sober. Maybe you're a little nervous about offering a toast—public speaking has that effect on many of us. But don't get tipsy in an effort to calm your nerves, Horn advises. "You need to present a good image, and you don't want to embarrass yourself," she says. "There's nothing worse than a drunk getting up and slurring his words."

Don't get *too* personal. We already suggested that you personalize your toast to the person or occasion. But don't overdo it. "Don't do or say anything that would be embarrassing to the person you're toasting," Horn says. "If there is some private matter that the recipient would rather keep private, don't put that in your toast." So, for example, if you are toasting a couple at a wedding reception, don't make cracks about the groom's prior conquests or the couple's future sex life. You risk embarrassing or offending them and their guests.

Avoid clichés. Avoid hackneyed phrases such as "down the hatch" when offering a toast, Horn advises.

Stay away from water. It's fine to toast with a nonalcoholic beverage as long as it's not water, Klinkenberg says. Water is supposed to bring bad luck, so an empty glass would be preferable if it comes to that.

Don't smash the glass. Some superstitions say that continuing to drink out of a glass after the toast dilutes the toast. Even so, don't follow the Russian custom of breaking a glass into the fireplace, advises Klinkenberg. Glass and crystal will melt and stick to the brick. Plus, smashing good crystal or a restaurant's glasses can bust your finances when you get the bill for damages.

When the Toast Is on You

One of these days—your wedding, your retirement, when you're named *Time* magazine's Man of the Century—you'll be on the receiving end of a toast. Here's how to handle it with grace.

Don't drink. Drinking when others toast you is akin to applauding yourself, Klinkenberg says.

Remain seated. It is inappropriate to stand while a toast is being offered to you, according to Klinkenberg. At a formal occasion,

> ## Toast through the Ages
>
> The practice of offering toasts began with the ancient Greeks, who had the quaint custom of spiking the punch with poison, according to Hilka Klinkenberg, managing director of Etiquette International. Offering a toast was considered a gesture of good faith.
>
> The term toasting comes from the Roman practice of putting a piece of burnt bread into the goblet to mellow the flavor of the wine. In England, toasted bread was placed in the bottom of the glass, and you drank until you reached it, Klinkenberg says.
>
> There are several theories as to how the custom of clinking glasses began. One, stemming from the Greek practice, says that by clinking glasses you could slosh the poison somebody may have placed in your wine back into theirs, Klinkenberg says. Another theory holds that the sound of clinking glasses was believed to drive the evil spirits out of the beverage, making it safe to drink.
>
> Toasting customs and traditions vary from one country to the next. In Korea, the glass is emptied and the last few drops are shaken out, then it is passed to the guest and the host refills the glass, Klinkenberg says. A glass is never refilled until it is completely empty in Korea. But in Japan, the glass is constantly refilled so it is never empty. The strongest and most formal traditions are found in eastern European, Germanic, and Scandinavian countries, Klinkenberg says.

however, the person offering the toast may ask you to stand with him, in which case you should, Horn adds.

Respond to the honor. Once the toast is finished, you should stand and, at the very least, thank the host for the generous gesture, Klinkenberg says.

Beat a Hangover

In the grand scheme of things, hangovers serve an important purpose. They are the price you pay for drinking too much. As the late English author Samuel Butler once noted: "It is immoral to get drunk because the headache comes after the drinking, but if the headache came first and the drunkenness afterwards, it would be moral to get drunk."

Morality aside, there is a very practical side to hangovers. And that's why you don't see scientists scrambling over one another to find a cure. "It's an ethical issue," says Carl Waltenbaugh, Ph.D., an immunologist at Northwestern University in Chicago. "Cure hangovers, and you remove a primary reason to curb your drinking."

Having one or two drinks a day has been shown to be good for your health. Having more than that—especially a lot more—clearly isn't. Still, it's a rare man who has never experienced those jackhammers in his head the morning after a night out. And on those rare occasions when that man is you, here's what you need to know.

Preventive Measures

Eat some honey. Whether it's spread on toast or a cracker, honey supplies fructose, which helps the body metabolize the alcohol ingested and reduces hangover symptoms, says Frederick G. Freitag, D.O., a spokesperson for the National Headache Foundation. Eat some before or after drinking.

Stick with the lighter stuff. There is anecdotal evidence suggesting that the congeners in dark-colored alcoholic beverages, which are the chemicals that give them their color and flavor, may promote a headache, says Alan Wartenberg, M.D., director of the addiction recovery program at Faulkner Hospital and assistant professor of medicine at Tufts University

School of Medicine, both in Boston. Red wine also seems to be a high-risk drink for the hangover-prone. Clear liquors such as vodka and gin are less cruel, although they can also make your head hurt if they're abused.

Be a sport. Sports drinks help restore sugar levels depleted by alcohol. "As nightcaps, they replace electrolytes and pump fluids in fast. The salt content helps your gut absorb fluids, which helps fight dehydration," says Dr. Waltenbaugh.

Go for bouillon. Drink a cup of bouillon or other liquid rich in salts and minerals that will help your body cope with dehydration, Dr. Freitag suggests. Plus, it's easy on your jumpy stomach.

Grab a cup of joe. A cup of coffee may offer some relief to your throbbing head and decrease the duration of the pain, Dr. Freitag says. Coffee can also make you feel edgier, however, so trial and error is the best course.

Get the NAC. N-acetyl-cysteine, an amino-acid supplement, replenishes your body with cysteine, which is a major component of glutathione (a powerful antioxidant). When glutathione is depleted, oxygen radicals damage tissues (hence, a hangover). More cysteine may help solve the problem. Research has been done only on mice, but some of Dr. Waltenbaugh's colleagues have seen their own symptoms clear up in 20 minutes from a few cysteine pills. Dr. Waltenbaugh recommends taking 500 to 1,000 milligrams of NAC when you are hung over.

Do not take NAC with acetaminophen. Use ibuprofen or aspirin instead for that hangover headache, Dr. Waltenbaugh says. Mixing NAC and acetaminophen may cause a dangerous reaction, he explains. Also, if you have a history of asthma or peptic ulcer, do not use NAC. If you take NAC at the recommended dose and experience nausea or severe vomiting, discontinue use and call your doctor.

Leave the acetaminophen on the shelf. Take aspirin or ibuprofen instead. "Acetaminophen can be very harmful to your liver when you drink," Dr. Waltenbaugh says.

Pick a Barber

One wonders: Does Don King go to a barber or a hairstylist? And would either one admit to it if he does? It's not exactly a question that will keep you up nights, but you may have wondered yourself whether you'd be better off with a barber or a stylist.

Wonder no more.

Traditionally, a cosmetologist's license required more hours of training than a barber's license, but that's changing. In many states, each license requires the same number of hours, but with a different curriculum.

Some hair professionals have licenses in both fields, says Rick Brockhoff, an instructor at the College of Hair Design, a barber and cosmetology school in Lincoln, Nebraska. "That would probably be the optimum person to go to," he says.

Some guys, however, aren't comfortable getting their hair cut in a salon, says Red Sidell, owner of Hanover Park College of Beauty Culture in Hanover Park, Illinois. For them, the all-male sanctuary of a barbershop may be best. But others prefer a woman cutting their hair, on the theory that they know what attracts the opposite sex.

Ultimately, the decision on which type of professional you chose to cut your hair comes down to simple personal preference.

Once you've decided whether to go to a barber or a stylist, you still have to find the right one. Try the following tips.

Ask around. Ask other guys—especially those with hairstyles that look great—who cuts their hair and if they are satisfied, Brockhoff advises.

Start off cautiously. "Usually the first time you go to somebody, you ask for a trim, just to be safe," Sidell says. "Then you get to know the person, you get a little confidence in him, and maybe you try something a little different."

Agree on your cut. One of the first clues is whether this barber or stylist is interested enough in you to ask questions about how you've been wearing your hair and whether you're satisfied with the way it looks, Sidell says.

If he doesn't ask, tell him how long you like your hair and what style you have in mind, Brockhoff says.

Conduct an interview. After all, this guy is applying for the job of cutting your hair. It's an important position, one that will affect how others view you. So make sure that you ask him how long he's been cutting hair, what his educational and training background is, and any other professional details you would request from someone who wants to work for you, Brockhoff suggests.

Show him some pictures. A lot of guys don't know layered hair from a layer cake. If you aren't sure how to describe the cut you want, show your haircutter a photo of the look you would like, or ask if he keeps a book showing different styles, Sidell suggests.

Look for detail work. A good barber or stylist not only makes what's on top look good, but he takes care of smaller details: trimming your eyebrows and that thicket of hair sprouting in your ears as well as cleaning up the fuzz on the back of your neck, Brockhoff says. When he's finished, he should use a hand mirror to let you see how the back of your head fared.

Don't be hasty. If the first haircut you get isn't perfect, don't give up on your haircutter too quickly. "Sometimes it takes a time or two for the person to get to know you and get it just the way you like it," Brockhoff says.

Cut it off. If, however, you get the sense that the guy with the scissors is about to make a mistake, don't be afraid to call off the cut. "If you know he's going a totally different direction than you are or you have the sense that he doesn't understand what you're saying, I wouldn't hesitate to say, 'I'm not comfortable with this. Maybe we should reschedule,'" Brockhoff says.

Look Stylish While You Sweat

Working out used to be simple for men. You threw on a T-shirt, jockstrap, gray shorts, sneakers, and baggy sweats and headed over to the local YMCA. There, you shot hoops, swam some laps, ran around the monotonous miniature indoor track until you lost count, or threw around some iron. It was a man's world.

That has all changed. Gyms today cater to women as well as men. They have more social events and classes on their calendars than the Love Boat, and more flashing lights, bells, and whistles than a disco. Which, in a way, is what fitness centers have become.

"There's no question that, in some cases, fitness centers are considered the singles' bars of today," says Paul M. Kennedy, Ed.D., area director for Bally Total Fitness in Phoenix and former head strength and conditioning coach at Rutgers University in Piscataway, New Jersey.

Even if you're not in the market for new love, exercising is a great way to socialize and even, heaven help us, network and do business. It's becoming quite common, says Dr. Kennedy, for an employer to make a workout at the gym or a round of golf a part of the process when scrutinizing prospective employees.

All of this means that it's no longer enough to work out so that you look better. You have to look better while you work out, too.

Exercising in Style

So what's the well-dressed man wearing to the gym these days? Glad you asked. Here are the answers.

Hang loose. Men, says Dr. Kennedy, sometimes fail to remember that they are 15 years older than they realize. They try to wedge into shorts that leave more crack exposed than an L.A. drug raid. Same with shirts. A tight tank top over a spare tire is just plain gruesome. "Most professional bodybuilders will tell you that they can always spot the amateurs in the room because they're the ones who wear the tightest clothing," says Dr. Kennedy.

Avoid polyester and acrylic. You really don't want to look like a refugee from K.C. and the Sunshine Band. Plus, these fabrics don't wick away sweat, which will leave you looking decidedly uncool. There are remarkable new microfiber garments on the market that breathe as well as look great.

As with anything, there are cheap versions and expensive versions. Go high-quality, says Anna Wildermuth, president and founder of Personal Images in Chicago and a certified image consultant. The pricier ones wear better and don't wrinkle. You can tell the difference by the feel. Good microfiber feels finer and softer, she says. A cotton blend—made with some manmade fibers—is the best because you want something that will absorb, breathe, and stretch.

Be solid. Don't wear anything with prominent slogans or logos, especially anything emblazoned with "Body by Budweiser." Solid, crisp colors are always in style, Wildermuth says. If you must wear a printed fabric, make sure it's a small, muted print.

Go vertical. "If you're a little bit overweight and tend to carry it around the middle, I wouldn't recommend horizontal striping," says Dr. Kennedy. It creates an illusion that you're even wider than you are.

Hawk the jewelry. Bracelets, bangles, gold chains, and rings are definitely a sports fashion no-no, says Wildermuth. A simple chain with a pendant is okay.

Know your area. "What may be acceptable in California may not be acceptable in the East," Wildermuth says. Generally speaking, the farther east you go, the safer you'll be dressing in conservative fitness attire.

Part Four

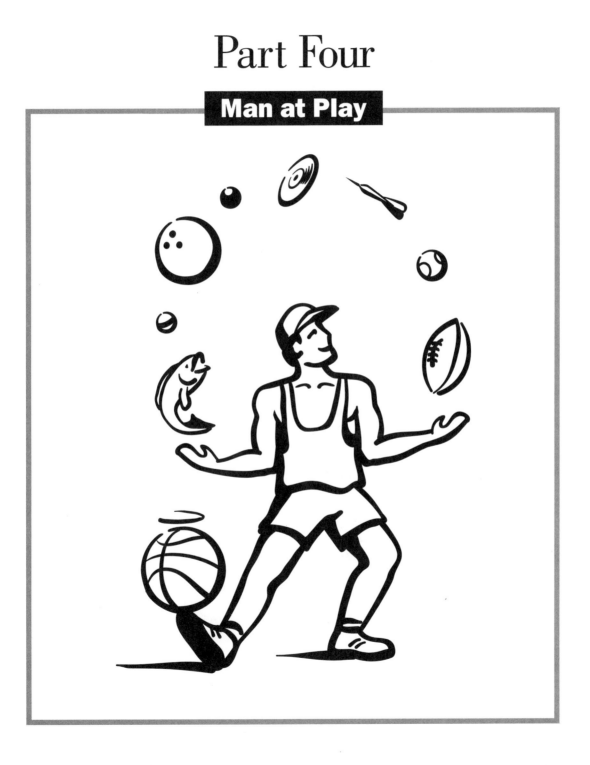

Win at Arm Wrestling

It conjures up images of the 98-pound weakling getting sand kicked on him at the beach: You get conned into arm wrestling some oaf, and he slams your arm down faster than you can say ouch. We feel your pain, so we went to Norm Devio, a five-foot-seven-inch, 150-pound physical education teacher from Brookline, Massachusetts, who has gotten the best of a few guys the size of NFL linemen. Devio has won seven national titles and about 350 trophies in arm-wrestling matches.

"I don't think you can ever overemphasize strength," Devio says. Strong fingers, hands, and wrists are most important. Devio trains two days a week, doing three sets of 8 to 14 repetitions in seven or eight exercises. Among them:

- Wrist curls. While seated, hold a dumbbell with your elbow locked against your inner thigh and your palm facing forward. Flex your wrist as far upward as it will go comfortably and then let it back down slowly. Repeat with your other hand.
- Reverse arm curl. Stand and grasp an easy curl bar or barbell with your palms facing backward and arms straight at your sides. Raise your arms upward while keeping your elbows snug against your body. Then let your arms down slowly. Devio tapes his easy curl bar or barbell handles to two or three times their normal thickness so that he can't touch his fingers to his thumb. He says this more closely simulates the position your hand is in while arm wrestling.
- Hammer curls. Sit at the end of a bench, knees bent, feet shoulder-width apart. Hold a dumbbell in each hand with your palms facing your body and arms

hanging down at your sides. Starting with the hand you use to arm wrestle, curl the weight up toward your shoulder as though it were a hammer you were lifting to drive a nail. Don't rotate your wrist. Keep your shoulders back and your back straight. You can alternate this exercise, first curling with your dominant hand, then with your other.

Devio practices with other guys on an arm-wrestling table once a week. Here are the techniques he uses to get the upper hand.

Get a grip. Devio and many other armed combatants keep their index fingers over their own thumbnails. Doing so raises the hand and wrist a little bit. "If you can get higher on another person's hand, you have an advantage in leverage alone," Devio says. Arm wrestlers must not, however, cover their own thumb knuckles when doing this grip. Elbows should be about 15 inches apart and form a triangle with you and your opponent's hands.

Arm yourself. For maximum leverage, keep your arm close to your body, Devio says.

Get a quick start. If the referee says "ready . . . go," Devio is generating tremendous torque on "ready." By this he means that he is already tensing his arm muscles as hard as he can, without pulling his opponent's arm. This expends about 75 percent of his energy, and on hearing "go," he releases the remaining 25 percent, at which time he will move his arm. "Outside of strength, there is nothing more important than that quick, fast start," he says.

Pull, don't push. Rather than trying to push your opponent's arm back at him, pull it or drag it sideways and hook it toward you, Devio says. This will open up his arm, causing him to lose leverage and possibly the match.

Roll him. Some arm wrestlers excel at a top roll in which they try to bend their opponent's hand back. A high grip is crucial. "Once you've lost your hands—unless you're incredibly strong—you've just about lost the match," Devio says.

Win an All-You-Can-Eat Contest

Ed "The Animal" Krachie attacks food with the pitiless swiftness of a lion felling a wildebeest. Twice he's won the Nathan's Famous Annual Hot Dog Eating Contest on Coney Island, setting a record—since broken—of 22½ dogs in 12 minutes.

In other contests, the six-foot-seven-inch, 350-pound mechanical engineer from Flushing, New York, has devoured 37 White Castle hamburgers in 10 minutes and a 5-pound roasting chicken in 2½ minutes. On national television, he bested a British sausage-eating champ by dispatching 10 hard-boiled eggs in 1 minute.

And, of course, there was the three pounds of Japanese ramen noodles he slurped down in 9½ minutes to win another title.

Unleashing "The Animal" Within

"I usually overwhelm the competition," Krachie says. What Krachie does isn't healthy—it's been estimated that he ingested three days' worth of calories and three weeks' worth of fat at the hot dog eating orgy—but clearly he is a man who knows a thing or two about winning all-you-can-eat contests. Here is his technique.

Don't fast. While you don't want to be full going into a competition, you shouldn't starve yourself beforehand, either, says Krachie. "I'll have dinner the day before, but I'll have it early, around three o'clock," he says. "When I get up, all I'll have is a bagel."

Keep your food moist. "I dunk my hot dog and bun in water," Krachie says. "You don't even taste the soggy bun." The moisture helps the food slide down your throat.

Condiments such as mustard or ketchup can help, but they also rob you of precious seconds while you apply them, Krachie says. Sipping water during a contest is a good idea, too—it was crucial to gulping down those 10 eggs in one minute, he adds.

Keep chewing to a minimum. "For the first eight or so hot dogs, I bite them in thirds and chew only a little bit and they go down," Krachie says. The more food you eat, however, the more you have to chew. "After you have 15 hot dogs, they don't want to go down any more. If you swallow a whole bite, it's going to come right back up. Chew when you have to."

Just remember: This is one "sporting event" where choking can cost you more than the win.

Ignore your competitors. Don't worry about whether the other guys are gaining on you. "It takes time away. When you're on such a fast pace, you need every second to concentrate on eating," Krachie says.

Stay focused. "Most people hit a wall after 12 to 13 hot dogs," Krachie says. "That's what separates the men from the boys. It's mind over matter." Even Krachie, however, concedes that an aching or queasy stomach is telling you that you have exceeded its limit.

Try different techniques. "A lot of other competitors can't use dunking, because it adds weight to the hot dog and they're already stuffed as it is," Krachie says. "Some people separate the hot dogs and buns and eat them separately. Some might take 10 tiny bites and swallow. This way they don't have to chew. Everybody has his own technique and all of these techniques have won before. Find something that works for you."

Remember: Size doesn't matter. Krachie eventually lost the Nathan's contest and his weenie-eating record to a teeny-weeny guy who's a foot shorter and 200 pounds lighter than him.

Throw a Perfect Spiral

Whether you're playing touch football or showing off for your kid, the ability to toss a pretty pass still ranks high in manly know-how. Plus it's just plain satisfying to throw a spiral so tight that Brett Favre would be impressed.

To learn how to throw a perfect spiral, we went to Jim Zorn, who passed for more than 20,000 yards in his 11-year NFL career. Zorn, who was the National Football Conference Rookie of the Year in 1976 and American Football Conference Player of the Year in 1978 with the Seattle Seahawks, also played for the Green Bay Packers, Tampa Bay Buccaneers, and the Canadian Football League's Winnipeg Blue Bombers before retiring in 1987.

Zorn is now the quarterbacks' coach for the NFL's Detroit Lions. But you don't have to be invited to training camp to benefit from his knowledge and experience. Consider this your own personal playbook. So pay attention, or we'll make you run laps.

Passing with Aplomb

Here are Zorn's step-by-step tips on how to pass like a pro.

Grip it good. Where a guy places his fingers on a football varies with the size of his hand, so find what is comfortable for you, Zorn advises. "If you have huge hands, you can probably grip it anywhere you want," he says. When he played, Zorn placed his ring finger between the third and fourth lace down on the ball, and his middle finger on the first lace.

More important is the placement of the thumb, Zorn says. It's the thumb that gives you a solid grip. Here's a quick way to see if you're holding the ball correctly: As you grip the ball, turn your passing hand over, palm up. You

should see enough daylight between the ball and your palm to wedge a finger in there. If the ball is resting flush against your palm, move your thumb farther back on the ball, Zorn says. Guys with smaller hands also should move their grip farther back on the ball, he adds.

Football Grip

Use two hands. Stand sideways to your target while watching him as you prepare to throw. If you are right-handed, your left hand should be placed on the front of the ball, Zorn says. Keeping both hands on the ball is especially useful to guys with small hands. "While letting it go, you only have to grip it with one hand for a very short time," Zorn says. Having both hands on the ball also prevents opening up your shoulders too quickly and dropping the ball too low. "You should hold the ball at the upper part of your numbers," Zorn says. "It should be back near your right shoulder if you are right-handed."

Put your best foot forward. Raise the elbow of your passing arm above shoulder height. As you step forward, release the hand on the front of the ball. Pivot your front foot so that it faces straight ahead. Both legs should be bent slightly. Pointing your front foot forward enables you to rotate your hips, which should occur simultaneously. At the same time, you should vigorously swivel your torso in the direction of the receiver, Zorn says.

Let 'er rip. The point at which the ball leaves your hand varies depending on the type of pass you throw, Zorn says. On a 15-yard sideline or comeback route, you might release it just forward of your head. If you're throwing a long bomb, the release will be sooner—perhaps a little to the rear of your head.

As you release the ball, your passing arm should go in a downward motion. "As you're pulling down, you want to feel a snap in your wrist and you want to throw your thumb down and out while you're releasing the football," Zorn says. The crispness with which your thumb leaves the ball enables you to get the nose of the football to fly level or slightly upward, starting its rotation and giving you a tight spiral and more control of the pass. Your arm should not be extended outward at the end of the pass. On the follow-through, your arm should come down near the middle of your body.

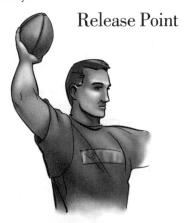

Release Point

Stay grounded. To ensure accuracy, you must keep your body balanced when you throw. The way to do that is to keep both feet on the ground during the passing motion, Zorn says. Unlike a baseball pitcher's follow-through, a quarterback remains almost upright with his knees bent, leaning forward slightly from the momentum of the throw.

Hit your receiver. Quarterbacks usually throw to the receiver, not a spot where they think a receiver will be, Zorn says. You should do the same. Once you've mastered the basics, you can try a fade route. This is where the quarterback lobs the ball to a corner of the end zone and hopes the receiver runs under it and catches it. You must lead the receiver, but it's not a conscious calcu-

lation as to where he will be, Zorn says. Like so many techniques in sports, you can get better at this with practice.

Passing Fancies

So who are the pro quarterbacks who threw the best spirals? We asked Babe Parilli, a quarterback for 16 years in the American Football League, the National Football League, and the Canadian Football League, whose last season as a pro saw him backing up Joe Namath when the New York Jets scored a stunning upset over the Baltimore Colts in Super Bowl III. In no particular order, here are Parilli's top five.

- **Dan Marino.** "He reads defenses quickly and makes decisions quickly. He does that probably better than anybody I've ever seen. Marino has an effective over-the-top spiral. He has a great touch and a quick release."

- **Joe Montana.** "Montana wasn't a very physical guy, but he probably had the greatest touch of all of them."

- **Dan Fouts.** "Fouts was tough and had a great presence. He just made things happen. He threw the ball a lot and was very productive, and he had the ability to put the ball between defenders."

- **Sonny Jurgensen.** "He threw it funny from the side, but his ball had probably the best spiral. He was very accurate."

- **Joe Namath.** "Namath was a lot like Marino. He had the quick release. He held the ball until the last possible second."

If he had to pick one quarterback as the best of the best, Parilli would choose Montana. The best quarterback he ever saw who wasn't a textbook passer? Bobby Layne. The best running quarterback ever? Steve Young. The most athletic quarterback? A tie between Steve Young and John Elway.

Pitch like a Big Leaguer

Pity the guy who regales his buddies or his kids with tales of his former pitching prowess—the Randy Johnson–like fastball and Roger Clemens–like slider with which he mowed down enemy hitters like weeds during his youth. He strides out to the park to provide the proof, and he's lucky if his heat would warm a ballpark hot dog bun.

You can still be a mound marvel even as your youth wanes, however. You simply need to vary your repertoire.

Throwing a Curveball

Nowadays, pitchers don't throw curveballs as much as they used to, preferring to rely on fastball and slider combinations, says Clyde Wright. He ought to know. Wright pitched 10 years in the major leagues, tossed a no-hitter, and won 22 games in 1970 with the Anaheim Angels. Wright—whose son, Jaret, is a talented big-league pitcher—now runs a pitching school in Anaheim, California.

"Curveballs are a lost art, and they shouldn't be," says Bert Blyleven, a Minnesota Twins broadcaster who pitched more than two decades in the major leagues, winning 287 games, striking out 3,701 hitters, and hurling a no-hitter. Blyleven cautions, however, that youngsters shouldn't throw curveballs because the stress could harm their still-developing arms. "I didn't start throwing a curveball until I was 14," adds Blyleven, who Wright and others say threw the best curveball they've seen.

Get a grip. Blyleven says he placed his index and middle fingers across the seams of the ball and his thumb along the seam below, where there is a horseshoe-shaped area. He

also kept his ring finger on the seam across from his thumb.

Curveball Grip

"That controlled the tightness of the rotation, and also the speed of the ball and the break of the ball," says Blyleven.

Hold the ball firmly. "If it's too loose, the ball has a tendency to slip out of your hand," Blyleven says. The shorter and tighter you want the ball to break, the firmer you grasp it.

Aim for the catcher's glove. "I never visualized the break of the ball," Blyleven says. "I visualized the end result. That, to me, was throwing the ball through the glove, not to the glove. It's almost like looking at a bull's-eye."

Make it snappy. Release the pitch when your arm is above your shoulder, rotating your wrist at the same time, Blyleven says. "You're pulling down with the torque of your arm motion, but you're also extending your arm and letting it follow through, creating the rotation or spin of the ball. Then you snap your wrist at the end."

Curveball Release Point

Hold back a bit. You don't want to throw the ball softly, but neither should you try to fire it as hard as a fastball, Wright says. "If you throw it really hard, it doesn't have enough time to turn over, to rotate. Therefore, it won't break as much."

Leg it out. Utilize your leg strength when you deliver the pitch, Blyleven says. Stand tall. Your legs should be in sync with your upper body. They should not fly open, and your torso should trail your legs when you are delivering the pitch. Blyleven says he shortened his stride by two to three inches when throwing a curve, which helped him keep up and over the ball. If you allow your fingers and wrist to rotate around rather than over the ball, the result will be a flat curveball.

Finish strong. The follow-through is crucial if you hope to keep the pitch low in the strike zone. High curveballs are often called hanging curveballs, and hitters crush them. That's because a hitter can see the entire ball when it's thrown at eye level, but as it drops lower, only the top half or so is visible, which makes it harder to hit, Blyleven says.

A right-handed pitcher should land with his left foot pointed toward home plate, Blyleven says. "To keep the ball rotating, you need a quick arm and a quick follow-through."

"When your pitching hand comes down, you should be able to see the palm of your hand in front of your chest," adds Wright. At the end of your momentum, your pitching arm should be outside your opposite knee, he says. If you finish with it inside your knee, you risk banging your elbow on the knee.

The Split-Finger Fastball

The splitter has become an increasingly popular pitch with major league hurlers, and it's easy to see why. "It looks like a fastball coming in, and it just drops at the last second," says Ross Grimsley, who won 20 games for the Montreal Expos in 1978 and 18 games for the Baltimore Orioles in 1974. "It's a very hard pitch to hit solidly." Grimsley's key pitch was a spitter, not a splitter, but as the former pitching coach for the minor league Reading Phillies, he has a working knowledge of all pitches.

The splitter can be hard on the shoulder and is not a pitch for kids to experiment with, Grimsley says. But if you're over the hill rather than a future king of the hill, read on.

Grip it good. Hold the baseball so that the place where the seams are the most narrow

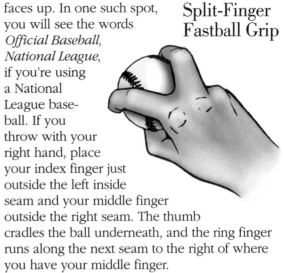

Split-Finger Fastball Grip

faces up. In one such spot, you will see the words *Official Baseball, National League,* if you're using a National League baseball. If you throw with your right hand, place your index finger just outside the left inside seam and your middle finger outside the right seam. The thumb cradles the ball underneath, and the ring finger runs along the next seam to the right of where you have your middle finger.

The pitch can be hard to master. "Usually, guys with big hands have a little bit easier time throwing it because they can split their fingers wide enough to where it will drop," Grimsley says.

Get down. Throw the splitter at the same arm speed as a fastball, Grimsley says. As with a curveball, you need to be on top of the ball—rotating your fingers and wrist over, not around, the ball.

Split-Finger Fastball Release Point

When you release the ball, snap your wrist straight down in a 12 o'clock to 6 o'clock motion, Grimsley says. You are not rotating your wrist as with a curveball, and on the follow-through, your palm should be facing down rather than pointing toward your body as with a curveball. Finally, the pitch must be released before your arm comes across your body on the follow-through motion in order to get the tumbling action on the ball.

Bowl a Strike

If the only strikes you've seen lately involve picket lines, maybe it's time to get some expert advice. That's what we did when we spoke to Dick Weber, a Hall of Fame bowler who has won 26 national and 6 senior titles and rolled 22 perfect games. Nowadays, Weber competes on the senior tour. He also puts on clinics and runs tournaments.

Before the Throw

Lighten up. Sometimes a 16-pound ball will make the pins fly in the air rather than into each other, Weber says. If this describes your game, consider using a lighter ball. "A lot of the pros now are using 14½- or 15-pound balls," he says.

Play the angle. A right-handed bowler with only a small hook would be wise to stand slightly right of center when he releases the ball, says Dick Ritger, a veteran instructor and operator of Dick Ritger Bowling Camps in River Falls, Wisconsin. A bowler with a sharp hook should stand left of center and angle the ball out to the right, he says. The degree to which a ball curves, however, can change from one lane to another and even on the same lane over the course of an evening as the amount of oil on it changes, Ritger explains.

Figuring out a lane's nuances is akin to judging a golf green, Weber says. "When you're warming up, you watch the break of the ball," he says.

Play it straight. Most bowlers do best when they keep their arm straight and close to their body on the back swing, Weber says. It should come up to shoulder level.

Pick your spot. On your path to the foul line, focus on the same spot each time before releasing the ball, Weber says. "A spot, whether it's at the foul line, 20 feet out on the lane, or 40 feet out, is like a gun sight." Don't focus on the pins.

Perfect your power step. The next-to-last step before the foul line is the one you push off on. A righty would use his right leg as the power step. "Your right knee is bent fairly well and it creates a nice slide forward on the left foot. The more the knee bends, the better off you are," Weber says.

The Throw

Get down. Release the ball at the bottom of your downswing. Your thumb should let go at about knee level. Shortly after that, gravity will take the ball from your fingers, Ritger says. If you let go too early or too late, you may lose velocity and bounce the ball.

Time it. Don't throw the ball too hard or too slowly. Doing so makes it less likely that you'll scatter pins widely, Ritger says. Your ball should travel 18 to 19 miles per hour and reach the pins in 2.1 to 2.2 seconds.

Throw the curveball. A right-hander's ball should curve from right to left. "You want the thumb coming out of the ball at a 10 o'clock or 11 o'clock position for a right-hander, and a 1 or 2 o'clock position for a left-hander," Weber says. "Then, from this release, you get a certain rotation that will make your ball curve."

Know your target. A right-handed bowler needs to lay the ball in the "pocket" between the one-pin and three-pin. For a lefty, it's between the one-pin and two-pin, says Weber.

Be a follower. On the follow-through, your hand should come up high—picture yourself reaching for the ceiling, Weber advises. A lazy follow-through lessens the rotation on the ball and hurts accuracy.

Pace yourself. Guys who are having a bad game often are rushing to the foul line and throwing the ball too hard, Weber says.

Make adjustments. The oil on lanes varies from one bowling alley to another, says Ritger. It can affect the break of your ball, so you need to adjust your game according to lane conditions.

Break at Pool

Here's one definition of humiliation: Some guy who thinks he's the next Willie Mosconi challenges you to a game of pool, you break, and the cue ball smacks the rack with all the force of a leaf floating to the ground. Compounding your shame, the only ball you sink is the cue ball. Scratch.

As one of only eight master billiards instructors in the world, Jerry Briesath can help. Here's his advice.

Be off-center. Professional pool players never place the cue ball in the center of the table. Why? The rack will spread better if the front ball is struck from an angle, says Briesath, who owns two billiard parlors in Madison, Wisconsin, and teaches the sport around the country. "They'll put it anywhere from a little off-center to way over near the rail," he says.

Stand and deliver. Stand up slightly higher when breaking than with other shots, Briesath advises. "You want to lift your head up 8 to 12 inches higher than normal, but still keep the cue level."

Build a big bridge. To generate power, your "bridge" on the break should be a couple inches longer than on other shots, Briesath says. If you are right-handed, the bridge is the distance from your left hand to the cue ball. Your left hand is your bridge hand. "A normal bridge would be 8 to 10 inches, so on the break, it is 10 to 12 inches," says Briesath.

Steady your stick. "If you lay your cue on the rail, you're as level as you can make it," Briesath says. This is critical because players often raise the butt end of the cue stick, causing the cue ball to hop and decreasing its power. Never put your bridge hand's thumb under the cue stick when you break from the rail; doing so will cause you to elevate your cue stick and will diminish your power.

Go slow. "The biggest gobbler of power is a fast backswing," says Briesath. "You have nothing left when you go forward." A fast backswing also hurts accuracy.

Don't be a spin doctor. Hitting the cue ball too high or too low decreases its speed and power. The trick to a good break is to put no spin on the cue ball. You do this by hitting it dead center. This also results in less movement by the cue ball after impact with the rack. "The less the cue ball moves after breaking, the more energy went into the rack," Briesath says. Plus, this leaves the cue ball near the center of the table and in better position for a follow-up shot.

Blast the front ball. The ball at the front of the rack is what you aim for on the break, and you should hit it smack in the center. If you fail, you are more apt to scratch and less likely to spread the balls well, says Briesath.

Play through. "A normal follow-through for a pro player on a regular shot is 4 to 6 inches past the cue ball," Briesath says. "On the break, you may want to go 10 to 14 inches past the cue ball."

Jump the jump shot. "Many novice players will say, 'I hit the cue ball so hard on the break that it jumps the table a lot,'" Briesath says. While it may impress your buddies, especially if you're on the third pitcher of beer, it's actually a sign that you're doing something wrong. "It has nothing to do with how hard you're hitting it. It's how badly you're hitting it," Briesath says. "Two things will cause a jump. The first is hitting that front ball on the side. The second is elevating the butt of the cue."

Keep your eye on the ball. Paying attention to where the cue ball goes after each of your breaks tells you how to correct it the next time, Briesath says. If, for example, the cue ball keeps veering to the left, aim a tiny fraction to the right on your next break. "The cue ball will tell you everything you need to know," he says. "Pros are always tweaking the break because they're using massive power and control is at its worst."

Throw Darts

Throwing darts looks so simple—stand about eight feet from a board and hit the bull's-eye. But how many players have you seen whose tosses resemble whiffle balls, fluttering futilely in flight en route to low scores? Roger Carter, an electronic components salesman from Doraville, Georgia, has no such problems. One of the best players in this country, he is on America's national team and for three straight years was the only American invited to compete in the international Embassy World Dart Championship in London.

Dart Pointers

Warm up. "You don't want to try to hit everything, because if you don't, you're going to get frustrated going into the tournament. I'll throw at the bull's-eye and just try to get a good rhythm going and get my aim down," Carter says.

Put your best foot forward. Stand at a right angle to the dartboard, right foot forward at the throw line if you are right-handed, advises Carter. If you're left-handed, go with the left angle and left foot forward. Don't, however, lean over the throw line trying to shorten the distance of your throw. "You're out of balance, out of control," Carter says. "You can't be consistent."

Hold it. Carter holds the dart above the knuckle on his thumb and below the knuckle on his index finger, with his ring finger resting on the point. He holds the dart about three-quarters of the length of the dart away from the point, near the shaft. "Whatever you find that works for you is the way you want to do it," he says. Once you find a grip that's comfortable, hold the dart firmly but don't squeeze it too hard.

Get the point. Keep the tip of the dart pointing toward the dartboard. Some guys throw darts with the tip facing up or down, but the darts are more likely to go higher or lower than they intend, Carter says. "If you hold it straight and you throw it straight, more than likely your dart is going straight where you're aiming."

Get set. Keep your forearm parallel to the dartboard as you are about to throw, Carter advises. Your upper arm should be still.

Find your release point. Bring the dart back toward your face before throwing. "I go right below my nose," Carter says. Since he's right-handed, the knuckle of Carter's right index finger grazes the lower right side of his mustache as he takes aim. Then he moves his arm straight forward, releasing the dart perhaps two feet forward from his face.

Be gentle. Using your arm only from the elbow to the wrist, toss the dart in an easy motion, Carter says. "You don't want to *make* it happen. You just want it to be natural." And don't try firing darts like a Randy Johnson fastball. "You lose control," Carter says. "The accuracy is not nearly as good."

Practice regularly. You won't be good at darts unless you practice, points out Carter. "It's not something where you can throw a few times and go out one night and expect to win. It takes a lot of time and dedication. If I can get 15 to 20 minutes in every day, I'm happy."

Join a league or enter tournaments. Winning a competition builds confidence, which is essential to playing well, Carter says. Don't get discouraged easily. "I played darts for 11 years before I started winning," he says. "I had patience. Now, I'm not afraid to play anybody."

Dress comfortably. During a tournament, Carter wears a shirt a size larger than normal to ensure freedom of movement. "If you like to tuck your shirt in, you may want to keep it out a little so it doesn't pull on you," he says. That doesn't mean dress like a slob, however. Serious dart players like Carter are trying to improve the game's image.

Win at Monopoly

Maybe you'll never be another Donald Trump. But with Monopoly, you can develop strategies that leave little to chance. "It's pretty much a luck-driven game," says Irvin Hentzel, Ph.D., professor of mathematics at Iowa State University in Ames, who has studied the game. "But with a little strategy, you can really increase your luck."

First, here are some things you should know, based on Dr. Hentzel's study.

- Illinois Avenue is landed on more than any other space. It's followed by Go, B.&O. Railroad, Free Parking, Tennessee Avenue, New York Avenue, Reading Railroad, and St. James Place, says Dr. Hentzel.
- Squares on the half of the board from St. Charles Place to Marvin Gardens get more action than those on the other half. The reason: When players go to jail, a full trip around the board is preempted.
- The orange monopoly properties have the highest return when $2,000 is invested in houses and hotels, says Dr. Hentzel. Expensive Boardwalk and Park Place are the second-best monopoly properties to own.

Here are some general strategies that will give you the edge in your quest to crush and humiliate your opponents.

Say "Buy, buy." Purchase as many properties as possible, because you need at least one monopoly to win, Dr. Hentzel advises. If you run short of cash, mortgage some of your acquisitions.

Know when to pay. If you go to jail and still need to buy properties, pay the $50 to get out right away. Otherwise, don't pay, suggests Dr. Hentzel.

Build smart. Don't put houses on your monopoly until you can afford to place three units on each property. With one or two houses, the rent is modest, but it jumps dramatically with three houses, Dr. Hentzel says. If you have two monopolies, build up one with at least three houses before you develop the second.

Call a reverse. Houses should be placed on properties in the reverse order from the direction of play, says Dr. Hentzel. This ensures that the property with the highest rent gets a house first. St. Charles Place rather than Virginia Avenue should get the second extra house on the magenta property, however, because it is landed on more often.

Make a trade. When trading properties, determine how much money your opponent has. If he's loaded, don't trade him a high-rent property, such as one of the greens, that will give him a monopoly. The opponent can then quickly build houses and clean you out, says Dr. Hentzel. Make the trade, however, if you can persuade him to include cash in the deal. This will leave him with too little money to build much right away, while giving you the capital to do just that.

Another scenario: Both of you have about equal sums of cash. Your opponent offers to trade you, say, Tennessee Avenue, for the more valuable Pacific Avenue, giving each of you a monopoly. Do it, says Dr. Hentzel. You will be able to put houses on your monopoly faster because they cost half as much.

Play as a peasant. If you have only $800 to $2,000 and doubts about whether you can build much on an expensive monopoly, follow a peasant strategy and go for a less expensive monopoly. The best bet is the orange properties, says Dr. Hentzel. Second choice: Boardwalk and Park Place. The latter cost a lot, but with only two properties needed for a monopoly, it can be done and the payoffs are huge.

Be a tycoon. If you're flush with cash, Dr. Hentzel suggests following his tycoon strategy. The best monopoly you can have now is the greens, he says. And remember to resist adding houses of your own until you can afford three on each site.

Play Frisbee with Your Dog

Looking for a way to meet women that's cheaper and less degrading than clubs and bars? Teach your dog to play Frisbee. You're in a monogamous relationship? It's fun anyway—for you and the pooch.

For pointers, we went to Peter Bloeme, director of the Alpo Canine Frisbee Championships. He has produced books and videos on Frisbee dogs through his Atlanta company, Skyhoundz. Bloeme won the World Frisbee Championships in 1976—a humans-only contest—then snatched the world canine title in 1984 with a border collie named Whirlin' Wizard. He and his hounds have performed at exhibitions throughout North America, Europe, and Japan.

Even if you're shy, playing Frisbee with a dog at a park is a great way to meet women. "It's a natural. I met a number of former girl-friends that way," Bloeme says. Eventually, he met his wife, a television producer, while pro-moting the championship contest.

Basic Training

Novices often think a dog should auto-matically catch a Frisbee and return it, Bloeme has found. "That's as silly as saying 'Heel' to an untrained dog and expecting the dog to heel," he says. "You have to break it down into a step-by-step process."

The following steps can be done in your living room or another confined area. You shouldn't start your dog's Frisbee training in a public place like a park—especially if he's a puppy—because he is likely to be distracted by other dogs there, Bloeme says. "Some dogs are going to be insanely focused on the disk from day one, and with others, you're going to have to develop that attention span," he adds.

Regardless of where you train, don't overdo it. Bloeme suggests 10 minutes three times a day for puppies and adult dogs just starting out. And he recommends starting slowly with easy tosses and jumps until your dog-athlete gets warmed up. Here's how to get started.

Introduce the dog to the disk. Throwing the Frisbee at your dog might simply scare him. Instead, put his food in the disk. Now, he's comfortable with it and associates it with something good. When he's finished eating, pick up the disk and put it away. Don't let it become a chew toy, Bloeme advises.

Shake, rattle, and roll. When your pup is feeling peppy—but not too soon after eating—take out the Frisbee and talk excitedly to him. He, in turn, will get excited, Bloeme says. Then, get down at your dog's level. Shake the disk and roll it a few times. When your pooch pounces on it, praise him.

Fake it. Still at your dog's level, fake tossing or rolling the Frisbee. After he starts to run for the disk, hold it out. When he returns and grabs it, give a tug to make sure he is grasping it firmly, then praise him. Repeat this step several times, Bloeme suggests.

Play catch. Position your dog directly in front of you—close enough that you almost can hand him the Frisbee. Now toss it to him. Praise him if he catches it. If he misses, don't let him pick it up. "The trick is not to chase after the Frisbee, but to catch it in the air," Bloeme says. "He only gets to keep it if he gets it in the air."

Advanced Training

Once your dog grasps the basic concept of catching the flying disk, the real fun begins. Here's how you can turn your pooch into a wonder dog.

Play fetch. Position your dog by your left side (if you are right-handed) and make the same sort of short toss you did in the basic training. The difference is that now your dog is moving to the disk, rather than having it come to him. If he catches it, praise him, as always. You've just completed your first real throw. Now, you can gradually extend the distance on subsequent tosses. Remember, your own ability is crucial to your dog's success. "If you don't throw well, he's not going to catch it," Bloeme points out.

Reel him in. If your dog isn't obedience-trained or is a puppy, chances are, he won't return the disk once he catches it. Dogs love to play keep away, and if you chase them, it just eggs them on, Bloeme says. To solve this, fasten a rope or cord to your dog's collar, and hang on to the other end. If your dog catches the disk and doesn't return it when you call him, give a sharp tug on the cord and say, "Come." Then reel him in and praise him. Don't punish your pet. "Then he won't want to come to you," Bloeme says. If you use this technique, be careful not to throw the Frisbee farther than the length of your dog's cord. "What will happen is, if you throw it too far, the dog gets his neck jerked back before he can catch the Frisbee," Bloeme says. "Basically, you're teaching the dog not to catch the Frisbee." If you realize you've thrown the disk too far, either let go of the cord or run along behind your dog, he suggests.

Take the leap. Until a dog is a year old, he should be allowed to leap only as high as he wants to, Bloeme says. After that, you can encourage him to soar higher. One way is to teach him the command "up" or "jump." Hold the disk over your dog's head. If he jumps up and takes it from your hand, say "up" or "jump." Then make short throws and bark the same command as he pursues the Frisbee.

Dog Day Afternoons

Every year, thousands of dogs and their owners compete in events leading up to the Alpo Canine Frisbee Championships, vying to become top dog.

"Any dog can be successful and enjoy the sport," says Peter Bloeme, director of the Alpo event. "It's a team sport, so it's not a question of getting the most athletic dog, because you could still fail."

Dogs enjoy running, jumping, and using their mouths, so playing Frisbee is naturally fun for them, Bloeme adds. "If an adult dog already chases balls and sticks, you can redirect him to the Frisbee. You can teach an old dog new tricks."

What types of dogs excel in competitions? Generally, those that weigh 30 to 65 pounds with average to above-average leaping ability that come from working-dog stock, Bloeme reports. Border collies, Australian shepherds, Labrador retrievers, and mixed breeds have been the most facile "disk jockeys," he says. Colleague Jeff Perry won the 1989 championship with a mutt he rescued from doggy death row at an animal shelter. The Michael Jordan of Frisbee dogs, however, was a whippet that took three world titles.

Whippet good.

Mix it up. Once your dog has become proficient at leaping, catching, and returning the Frisbee, you can introduce other throws: sidearm, overhand, wrist flip, skips, between your legs, behind your back, and multiple rapid-fire tosses, if you're able to, Bloeme says.

Patience is the key. Even a pro like Bloeme says it can take him anywhere from five minutes to teach a dog all the steps to one week for each step. "Frisbee with dogs is not a science," he says.

Win at Poker

In 1989, when he was in his midtwenties, Phil Hellmuth Jr. won the World Series of Poker in Las Vegas, and with it, $750,000. "Not bad for four days' work," he chuckles. In his first nine years as a professional poker player, Hellmuth, of Palo Alto, California, already has risen to third all-time in World Series of Poker winnings, with more than $2 million. Combine that with his take in other tournaments, and he has pocketed more than $4 million for knowing when to hold 'em and when to fold 'em.

"Poker is a pretty nice way to make a living," says Hellmuth. "There's a lot of money in it."

Play Smart

If your livelihood depends on the luck of the draw, this chapter won't help you much. But if achieving poker parity with your buddies will restore some wounded pride, read on. Hellmuth estimates that poker is 60 percent skill and 40 percent luck, so you can improve your game. Here's how.

Do the math. "The math part of poker is very simple," Hellmuth says. Say, for example, that you are playing five-card draw and are dealt four spades. You know that of the other 47 cards in the deck, nine are spades, giving you almost a one-in-five chance of drawing one more for a flush. Add to that the knowledge that a flush will win most hands, and clearly it behooves you to place a bet and ask for one more card. Usually.

The pot should contain at least five times the amount it will cost you to draw a card, writes the late gambling expert John Scarne in *Scarne's New Complete Guide to Gambling.* So if the opening bet was $1, there must be $5 or more in the pot before it's worth your risk to pay $1 for another card.

Be disciplined. "The gambler who plays a lot of hands almost always loses," Hellmuth says. "You need discipline to throw away the weaker hands." Scarne recommended dropping out immediately if you aren't dealt a pair or better, or a four-card flush or straight. Also keep in mind that the more people playing, the harder it is to draw the cards you need. So if you have a pair of jacks, you may realistically hope to draw a third if it's just you and a buddy playing. But the odds are much lower if it's you and a half-dozen other guys.

Stick to your strategy. Don't deviate from your game plan, advises Hellmuth. If your strategy is to bet only a few hands, don't start playing every hand once you are in a losing streak in an attempt to reverse it. Chances are you'll only compound your problems because now you will be betting on hands that have little likelihood of winning.

Take a break. If you hit a streak where every hand you're dealt stinks, take a break, Hellmuth suggests. Use the bathroom. Go for a short walk. "It just calms people down to be away from it for a few minutes," he says.

Don't become overconfident. Players sometimes hit a hot streak—called a rush in pro poker parlance—in which they win almost every pot. If you should be so lucky, don't think you're invincible and start betting low-percentage hands. Your rush will fizzle quickly, Hellmuth says.

Being a Real Player

Knowing the cards isn't enough. You also have to know who's holding them. So it pays to study your opponents. Here are some things to look for.

File under "Bluffing." Hellmuth thinks he's one of the best at knowing when a player is bluffing. Here's the sort of thing he looks for.

One of the players, in a show of confidence, tosses his chips in the pot with extra gusto—only to be called and discovered bluffing. "I would look for him to repeat that action. I wouldn't call it to his attention, or he could use it deceptively against you.

"A lot of times people give something away when they're talking," Hellmuth says. "Most of the time in an amateur game, when someone is talking, they have a strong hand. They spend a lot of energy trying to sell their hand to you." If you only play nickel-and-dime poker games, don't bother trying to read bluffs, Hellmuth adds. With such low stakes, most players will wager aggressively regardless of the hand they're dealt.

Be consistent. The same things that can enable you to read a player's bluff can also be used against you. "I would be consistent," Hellmuth says. "If I successfully bluffed a hand and I remembered how I made the bluff and I noticed people paying attention to it, I would try to repeat that same motion and action later when I wanted somebody to call me."

Wager wisely. Knowing the tendencies of your fellow poker players is key to betting wisely, says Hellmuth. Let's assume you are dealt a very strong hand. If your colleagues are mostly conservative card players who don't play many hands, you don't want to bet aggressively, because they'll fold and you'll win little money. If a couple of your opponents seldom fold, then bet hard because they'll probably stay in and jack up the amount of the pot to a higher amount than five conservative players would, Hellmuth says.

Check-raise occasionally. One way to ensure that your cautious colleagues don't fold too quickly when you have a strong hand is to check-raise—decline to bet when it's your turn, but then call and raise when somebody else does, Hellmuth says. It's also a great way to bluff your opponents, because it's commonly

Odds Are

The late gambling expert John Scarne computed the odds of drawing various hands in poker in his book *Scarne's New Complete Guide to Gambling*. Following are some of his findings.

Chances of improving your hand in draw poker when you've been dealt one pair and are drawing three cards:

- **Odds against any improvement: 2½ to 1**
- **Odds against making two pairs: 5 to 1**
- **Odds against making three of a kind: 8 to 1**
- **Odds against making a full house: 97 to 1**
- **Odds against making four of a kind: 359 to 1**

Chances of improving your hand in draw poker when you've been dealt three of a kind and are drawing two cards:

- **Odds against any improvement: 8½ to 1**
- **Odds against making a full house: 15½ to 1**
- **Odds against making four of a kind: 22½ to 1**

assumed that the player employing a check-raise has a good hand, says Hellmuth. This, in turn, scares a lot of players into folding.

Don't dwell on the money. If you constantly fret about the money while you play, it can distract you from what you should be doing—following a strategy, observing your opponents, and doing the mental math to make good bets, Hellmuth says.

Don't play over your head. "If you're playing in a game you can't afford, that means you can't take a loss in it without it hurting you," says Hellmuth. That gives your well-heeled opponents an advantage. "They can afford to win and lose, and they can smell the fear on you. They might bet all their chips with nothing, because they know you're afraid to call."

Win at Carnival Games

A walk along a carnival midway is akin to a stroll through an outdoor gambling casino. Instead of tuxedo-clad croupiers and dealers separating you from your money, there are carnies in T-shirts and tattoos doing the same thing.

Carnival games aren't a good gamble because those with big prizes are difficult or impossible to win. Some games are easy to win, but the prize costs much less than what you paid to play. And some games are rigged, though the industry is improving, says Bruce Walstad, a detective with the Franklin Park, Illinois, police department, whose job includes investigating carnival games and who conducts workshops on the subject for law enforcement officials. Here's what you should know if you're trying to win at carnival games.

Observe others. Before playing, "watch somebody else play the game and try to judge its difficulty," advises Walstad.

Learn the rules. Even when you think you've won a prize, a carny may thwart you by saying that you crossed the foul line or violated another supposed rule, Walstad says. Ask about the rules up front.

Hit it big. Carnivals at large venues such as state fairs are generally more reputable than small outfits that pop up in, say, a shopping center parking lot, Walstad says.

Stand up for yourself. If you really believe that you have been cheated by a carnival game operator, complain to a police officer patrolling the area, Walstad says. Or find the carnival owner. "Generally, they will come up with some sort of compromise," he says.

Best Bets

Unless you're wearing a T-shirt that says "Sucker," you should go to a carnival to have fun, not to strike it rich. That said, some games offer better odds of winning than others. Here's a tip sheet.

Group games. "Group games, where you're not playing against the house but against other players, are generally excellent to play," Walstad says. That's because with several players paying to play each time, the carny has no need to cheat you out of an inexpensive prize. Examples of group games include water races played with squirt guns, such as shooting water through a clown's mouth to fill up a balloon atop his head, and Derby, in which players advance their race horse to the finish line by returning a ball through various slots in a pinball-like device. Prizes may be modest, but every contest has a winner.

Hi-striker. This is the old carnival staple in which the player swings a big mallet and tries to drive a metal cylinder to the top of a wire track, where it rings a bell. Like any game, it can be rigged, but there is no need to, Walstad says. "You pay $1 to hit that thing to show your strength in front of your buddies or your girlfriend. If you win, you get a 50-cent prize. And the more that bell clangs, the more people are going to come over and play the game."

Bust three balloons. Games in which you pay for three darts and try to pop balloons are generally aboveboard, says Sherry Hopkins, division administrator with the Department of Inspections and Appeals in Des Moines, Iowa, whose job includes overseeing carnival games. Sometimes, however, balloons may be underinflated or the darts dull, making it harder to pop them, she says.

Glass pitch. You toss coins or Ping-Pong balls at glasses, ashtrays, and the like. If the coin or ball stays in an item, you keep it. The glass pitch is neither rigged nor hard to win, writes Gene Sorrows, a former carny who exposed many of his brethren's secrets in a book titled *All about Carnivals*, published by the American Federation of Police.

Milk can game. Toss a softball into a dairy milk can that has a smaller than normal opening on top, and you win a large stuffed animal. It's difficult, but the game is not rigged, Sorrows writes.

Gullible Gambles

"There's a sucker born every minute," P.T. Barnum, the legendary showman, is reputed to have said. The following games are living proof.

Conversion chart games. Any carnival game in which you accumulate points whose worth is interpreted by a carny holding a conversion chart is a loser. "There is no way you're ever going to win," Hopkins cautions.

Shooting hoops. The basketballs may be slightly overinflated or deflated, or the hoop could be oval-shaped rather than round, Hopkins points out.

Six cat. You must knock three stuffed cats off a shelf with a like number of baseballs. In some games, the cats are wedged so tightly atop the shelves that they are hard to topple. Dishonest operators arrange the canvas at the rear of their tent so that it touches the cats and keeps them from falling off the shelf, Walstad says. Others have been known to operate a hidden foot pedal connected to a rod, which catches the falling feline and prevents it from toppling off the shelf.

One ball. The player tries to spill three milk bottles in a pyramid from their stand by throwing a ball. Sometimes one or more of the bottles is so heavy or the ball you're given is so light that it's impossible to do, Walstad says. A carny may demonstrate how easy this game is by placing one heavy bottle atop two light bottles. Then he throws the ball at the two light bottles on the bottom, and all three come tumbling down. "If you're going to play that game, ask to feel the weight of the bottles," Walstad advises.

Carny Lingo

Deciphering carny conversations can be as baffling as listening to your crazy Aunt Agnes. Some translations, courtesy of *All about Carnivals* by Gene Sorrows:

Flash. The prizes on display in a game booth.

Flat store. A rigged game.

Gaff. The device used to rig a game.

Hanky pank. A game that's easily won, but the prize is really cheap.

Lot lice. Customers who hang around the midway without spending money.

Mark. A person playing carnival games. Any outsider. You.

Plush. Stuffed animals that are prizes.

Punk ride. A kiddie ride.

Rag. A small stuffed item in a plastic bag given out in large quantities as prizes at some games.

Slum. Inexpensive prizes such as whistles and plastic rings.

Stick. A carny who pretends to be a mark who wins a game.

Bushel baskets. The rules usually call for the player to lob two softballs into a bushel basket. If both stay in, he wins a prize. As a come-on, a carny may take two balls and toss them in a basket. Only thing is, he's standing on the other side of the counter where it's a shorter throw and the balls are less likely to bounce out, Hopkins says. Ask him to demonstrate the game from where *you're* standing.

Another trick: After the carny makes his first throw, he leaves the ball in the basket. This cushions the second ball when it lands in the basket, preventing it from bouncing out, Hopkins says. But if a player manages to get his first ball to remain in the basket, the carny will casually remove it before the player makes his second toss.

Clean a Fish

It's a dirty, smelly job, but there are good reasons to clean your own fish. "If you're really concerned about the way you're going to present the fish, the way you're going to cook it and eat it, nobody's going to exhibit more care with it than you are," says Ken Schultz, a staff writer for *Field and Stream* magazine who has been an avid fisherman for 28 years, has cleaned several hundred fish, and is writing a sport fishing encyclopedia.

Before you start, here are two things to keep in mind.

Use a good knife. Generally, you should use a sharp knife with a moderately thin, flexible blade, Schultz says. For smaller species, however, you can even make do with a sharp pocket knife. If you are inexperienced at cleaning fish, don't use an ultra-sharp instrument, he cautions. You could inadvertently demolish some of the meat that you're trying to carve.

Take proper care of the fish. Don't leave fish you have caught lying in the bottom of the boat, exposed to the sun, grime, and gasoline fumes, Schultz says. Keep fish on ice, or left hanging in the water on a stringer. Tackle stores sell several varieties of stringers that have easy unsnappable loops designed to hold your catch through its lower jaw or gills.

Gutting

Unless you're filleting a fish, you will be removing the scales and the entrails. Here's how.

Scrape the scales. Don't use the same knife you will be employing to gut the fish—you will dull it, Schultz says. There are special de-scaling instruments sold for this job, or you can even drag the inner spoon edge of a tablespoon against the grain of the scales until they are shed, Schultz says. If possible, remove the scales in a sink with cold running water to minimize getting them all over everything.

Get the scoop. To open up the fish, cut along the entire length of its belly starting at the anal vent, which is just in front of the tail. Cut from there to just below its head, making a vertical slit where you stopped, Schultz says. Then pull back on the gills and cartilage in the neck area to expose the entrails, and scoop them out. You will need to scoop out the entire body cavity, all the way to the end, to get them all out.

Cut off its head. Some people prefer to leave the head on a fish, but if you want to remove it, start your cut behind the pectoral fins—the fins before the gills—and cut through the fish on an angle toward the head. With larger fish, you may have substantial backbone that is tough to cut through. Use a larger, sturdier knife than you would on a smaller fish, Schultz says.

Go for two scoops. Scoop inside the belly incision to retrieve any remaining matter in the body cavity, particularly scraping along the backbone. The backbone runs for the length of the body about one-third of the way down from the top of the fish.

Rinse. Once you've finished, rinse the fish in cool, clean water inside and out, Schultz advises. This will cleanse it of blood and tissue that you don't want mixing with the meat.

Steak your claim. Large fish can be cut into steaks. Starting below the head and working your way to the tail, make uniform cuts of ¾ of an inch to 1½ inches, Schultz suggests. Cut across the side of the fish, through the backbone, and out the other side. "One inch, give or take a little, is an ideal size."

Filleting

If you divide the fish into two lengthwise layers, known as filleting, you are limited to panfrying, grilling, or broiling it. On the other hand, you needn't gut the fish, and it removes all bones from most species if done right.

"Bones disturb some people," Schultz notes. Here's how to fillet.

Decide how you want to cook it. If you leave the skin on, you will need to scrape off the scales before you start. "For grilling or deep-frying, you need to leave the skin on to hold the meat together. Otherwise, most people want to cut it off to avoid the fatty tissue, which is where possible contaminants are stored," Schultz explains.

Make the cut. Lay the fish on its side, head to the right, tail to the left. Enter behind the pectoral fin, on the angle of the gills. You will be making one long incision, starting behind the pectoral fin and moving toward the head, turning direction, then slicing down the length of the body and ending at the tail. Cut into the body until you hit backbone, Schultz says.

The Ones That Didn't Get Away

You think that 5-pound trout you caught is a mess to clean? It could be worse. The largest officially ratified fish ever caught on a rod was a 16-foot-10-inch, 2,664-pound great white shark on a 130-pound test line in the waters off South Australia in 1959, according to *The Guinness Book of Records*.

A great white shark weighing 3,388 pounds was caught in 1976 off Western Australia, but the catch is unratified because whale meat was used as bait.

At the other extreme, the smallest freshwater fish in the world would be decimated if you tried to clean it. The dwarf pygmy goby, found in streams and lakes in the Philippines, ranges from little more than one-quarter of an inch to a tad more than one-third of an inch in length.

Cutting to the Backbone

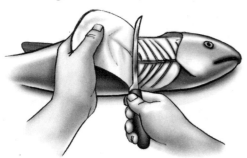

Reverse direction. At the backbone, while still inside the fish, twist the knife clockwise until it is facing the tail. The knife should be flat now, directly against the backbone. Slide it down the length of the vertebrae all the way to the tail. Don't be afraid to cut right up against the backbone—but not through it. Beginners often make this mistake, especially on a smaller fish, Schultz says.

Skin it. Flip the fillet over, hold on to the tail, and slip the knife between the skin and the meat, starting at the tail. Keep the knife slightly angled toward the skin, while sliding it from the tail end to the head.

Rib it. The remaining bones are the ribs. Start your slice underneath these bones and cut out this entire section, again keeping the knife as close as possible to the bones.

Slicing a Clean Fillet

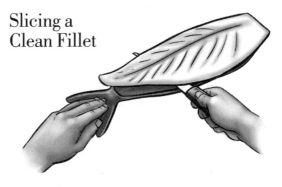

Repeat and rinse. Turn the fish over and repeat the same procedure on the other side. When all is done, don't forget to thoroughly rinse the fillets in cold water.

Shoot a Free Throw

Okay, there's no way you have the stuff to dunk like Michael Jordan or sky for a rebound like Dennis Rodman. But even if you have the moves of a bricklayer rather than a ballplayer, there is one thing you can excel at on a basketball court: shooting free throws. Here's how.

Toe the line. Stand behind the foul line dead center in front of the basket, says Buzz Braman, who has tutored numerous NBA players and is known in hoop circles as The Shot Doctor. On a hardwood court, you can do this by finding a nail that marks the exact center of the foul line. A right-handed shooter should line up his right foot with the nail, with his left foot trailing, says Braman, who once made 738 consecutive free throws, and 1,121 out of 1,144—98 percent—in a one-hour exhibition.

Get in a routine. Bounce the ball several times to get a feel for it, suggests Al Masino, a former NBA player and camp director of the Al Cervi and Al Masino Basketball Camp in Rochester, New York. This also is a relaxation mechanism, Masino says. Bounce the ball the same number of times every time you go to the foul line, so that you develop a routine.

Focus on the front of the rim. Visualize a match tip located there, and if you shoot the ball just over it, the match will light, Masino says.

Bend your knees. "You get your power from your legs," Masino points out.

Keep your elbows close to your body. "You shouldn't be like a chicken and have them out to the sides," says Masino.

Go to L. As you raise the ball to the shooting position, your shooting arm should form an L, Braman says. Master this, and you will never miss a free throw to the left or right of the hoop.

Assume the position. If you are right-handed, place your left hand on the side of the ball to prevent it from falling off the L and to guide the ball into the shooting position, Braman says.

Block out. Be mentally tough, Braman says. "That means focusing in and blocking things out."

Watch your finger. In one easy motion, release your guide hand from the ball and snap the wrist of your shooting arm toward the basket. When you release the ball, your fingers should be facing the basket. The shot should roll off your fingertips to give the ball backspin. At no time should the ball be resting in the palm of your shooting hand. The three fingers most critical to guiding the ball toward the basket are the thumb, index finger, and middle finger, Masino says.

The ball should leave your index finger last. "Wherever your index finger points to on the follow-through is where the ball goes," Braman explains.

Shoot the ball in an arc. Masino suggests visualizing yourself in a telephone booth trying to shoot through the top of the booth, not through the sides.

Follow through. When you release the ball, your shooting arm should be fully extended with your wrist down, Braman says. Your hand and fingers on the follow-through should be flat in the shape of a swan's head, adds Masino.

Don't twist. After taking the shot, the fingers on your guide hand should be extended and still facing where the ball was, Braman says. Most players have their guide hand facing the basket on the follow-through, which means they twisted their hand and pushed the ball off course, he says.

Be on your toes. Your follow-through should find you standing on your toes, Braman points out.

Part Five

Man at Work

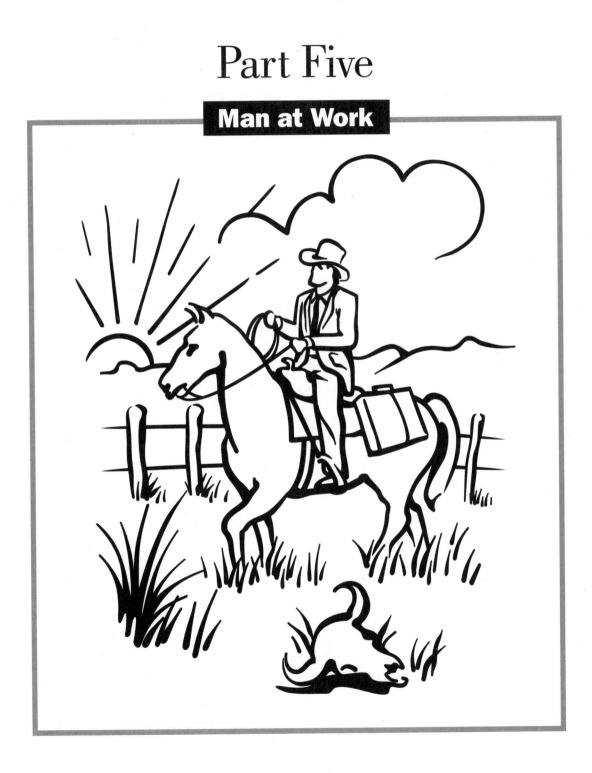

Play Hooky Guilt-Free

You know the feeling. You wake up one weekday and you just don't feel like going to work. You hate your job. Or you like your job, but you're a little burned out. Or it's a gorgeous day and you'd rather be fly-fishing, body surfing, or napping in a hammock. And so you decide to phone in "sick" and—being the honest, conscientious worker you are—agonize over feigning an illness. "I would guess that a significant minority, if not a majority, of workers do that," says James Campbell Quick, Ph.D., professor of organizational behavior at the University of Texas at Arlington and editor of the *Journal of Occupational Health Psychology*. It's commonly called a mental-health day. We're here to say that you have no reason to feel bad about taking one.

If your body breaks down and you get a cold or the flu, nobody thinks twice if you take a day or two off from work. But if you want a day away to replenish your emotional and spiritual energy, your boss may view you as warily as the latest expense report you submitted.

Your emotional and spiritual health, however, is just as important as your physical health, Dr. Quick says. "We need to balance the efforts of working, which is a necessity to provide for the things we need in life, with recovery time to care for ourselves—to replenish our supplies of energy and rejuvenate ourselves."

The ethical dilemma for some workers, however, is that they hate being forced to lie and claim they have an illness, says Nan De-Mars, founder and president of Executary Services, an organization that offers workplace ethics seminars in Minneapolis, and author of *You Want Me to Do What?: When, Where, and How to Draw the Line at Work.*

The European Solution

If you feel guilty about phoning the office with a phony rasp in your voice, don't despair. Guilt is a good thing, according to Dr. Quick. "When we feel guilty about an action that we have engaged in, that should help prevent us from engaging in that action again," he says. Should we feel guilty about skipping work when we're healthy? That depends, perhaps, on whether we really do need a day off to recharge our brain cells. "We need to be able to argue with ourselves about whether what we're feeling is warranted and legitimate," says Dr. Quick.

Still feel guilty? Then remember this: A lot of workers in other developed countries, such as in Europe, get more vacation time than most of us. Americans, on average, get 10 vacation days a year, or two weeks. No wonder your brain feels like oatmeal some days.

If you lived in Sweden, it might be different. Workers there receive an average of 30 vacation days—six weeks—annually. In France, the average is 25 days, and in Britain, 22 days. Germans also fare much better than Americans—they get an average of 18 vacation days.

You can take some solace, however, in the fact that the Japanese, like us, get an average of 10 vacation days per year. And pity the poor worker in Mexico—he gets an average of 6 vacation days, or barely more than a week off.

Taking Your Time

If you hate saying that you're sick when you aren't, try broadening your definition of what sick means. "One of the reasons you're taking a mental-health day is that you're out of gas, emotionally and psychologically," says Dr. Quick. "You could say that at one level you are legitimately sick. So the day off becomes one of recovery and rejuvenation."

Here are some strategies that experts say

can help you get the day you need without jeopardizing your job.

Plan ahead. Ask for a mental-health day off well in advance of when you'll need it. If you are about to tackle a difficult, time-consuming project with a deadline in, say, four months, ask at the onset for the day off after the deadline, says DeMars. A boss who knows you are taking on a big workload is less likely to begrudge you a day to decompress afterward.

Consider telling the truth. Yeah, we know it sounds crazy. But it just might work. When you call in sick, simply say you are fatigued and are taking a day off to rejuvenate yourself. But do so only if you have a good feel for how your employer might take this, advises DeMars. "Most men would never admit they need a mental-health day," she says. "It's perceived as wimpy."

Take a vacation day. This one's a tough choice. With so few vacation days available to most workers, it's understandable that they hate the idea of squandering one. But it is a way to avoid lying when you need a mental-health day, says DeMars. That way you needn't mention more specifically why you are taking the day off.

Be ready to work. Regardless of whether you are candid or deceptive about the true reason you take a day off work, come back the next day enthused and productive, DeMars says. You'll feel better about your having taken the day off, and your boss will, too.

Benefit from an enlightened company. If you still feel conflicted about phoning in sick for a mental-health day, consider working for a company that doesn't divide time off into vacation and sick days. Some firms simply give employees what is called personal time off (PTO), rather than vacation and sick

days. Employees get a certain number of days off, depending on their length of service. They can take them for any reason, so there is no need to explain why they are taking a day off. This seems to be a growing trend, DeMars says.

"What it's doing is putting into the hands of the employees the discretionary control to decide how to use that resource," says Dr. Quick. "That's a good thing."

Be an advocate. "Try to make a change within your company," suggests De-Mars. "Bring the issue up so maybe the company will consider some of your sick days as mental-health days."

Sick Excuses

Forget the ethical dilemma about whether to call in sick when you're not. You're in a quandary because you've already used the cold and flu and migraine headache excuses. Now, you're ready to take another mental-health day and you're frantic because you've run out of stories to spin. Here are some creative excuses we found on various Internet sites. Use them at your own risk.

- **Constipation has made me a walking time bomb.**
- **The dog ate my car keys. We're going to hitchhike to the vet.**
- **I just found out that I was switched at birth. Legally, I shouldn't come to work knowing that my employee records may now contain false information.**
- **If it is all the same to you, I won't be coming in to work. The voices told me to clean all the guns today.**
- **The psychiatrist said it was an excellent session. He even gave me this jaw restraint so I won't bite things when I am startled.**
- **I can't come in to work today because I'll be stalking my previous boss, who fired me for not showing up. Okay?**

Get Ahead without Being a Suck-Up

Most of us have observed with chagrin the meteoric rise of a colleague who is a sycophant—a bootlicking, obsequious lackey whose toadyism seemingly has netted him a promotion or a pay hike that somebody else deserved more. Somebody like us.

Must a man shed all vestiges of self-respect to advance in the working world? No, say workplace consultants. Here's how to get ahead and still be able to look yourself in the mirror.

Be a company man. "The best way to influence your boss is to use his self-interest and not yours," says Alan Weiss, Ph.D., president of Summit Consulting Group in East Greenwich, Rhode Island. "In other words, focus on your contribution to the company, not on what you're doing. It's one thing to say, 'I show up every day on time.' But to say, 'Our sales increased 2 percent last month because of the new procedure I introduced'—that's different."

Keep calm. Discuss your request in the same calm tone of voice you would use to discuss a strategy for an upcoming sales conference, Dr. Weiss advises. "It should never be with your hat in your hand, nor should it be demanding. It should be colleague to colleague, a credible discussion of the merits of the case."

Time it right. Most people wait until their annual job evaluations to tout their accomplishments to their bosses, Dr. Weiss says. By then, those achievements may be a blur in your boss's memory. Instead, send your boss a memo detailing your achievement soon after each major accomplishment, he suggests.

Increase your load. Take on an extra project or two and the responsibilities that come with it, advises Robert Vecchiotti, Ph.D., president of Organizational Consulting Services of St. Louis. A person is likely to be given a salary bump only because he is given additional responsibilities, he says.

Take the initiative. Look for tough issues to solve before they are evident to others, says Dr. Vecchiotti. "If you're prepared with a good analysis of the situation and a couple of options, you'll attract attention. That's what really distinguishes people who are going to move quickly and get raises as a consequence."

Become indispensable. If you have knowledge, skills, or abilities that others in your company don't possess, you increase your bargaining power, says Michael Mercer, Ph.D., an industrial psychologist with the Mercer Group in Barrington, Illinois, and author of *How Winners Do It: High Impact Skills for Your Career Success.* "The more replaceable you are, the less leverage you have."

Be vague. If you're seeking a pay raise, don't specify how much, Dr. Weiss advises. "You might ask for 8 percent, but it could be they were prepared to give you 20 percent," he says. "Nobody ever negotiates upward."

Career Killers

Just as there are things you can do to increase your chances of winning a raise or promotion, there are surefire steps to sabotage your career. Here's how to avoid three of the most common mistakes.

Stay out of politics. If you have the political instincts of a 10-term congressman, feel free to delve into the backbiting world of office politics. If not, stay on the sidelines. "If you play on somebody else's ball field with his equipment and his rules, you lose," Dr. Weiss says. "Stay above the fray. Never try to elevate yourself by degrading someone else."

It may seem that being a political animal is essential to advancing your career, but you can turn your indifference to your advantage, Dr. Weiss says. "Point out that you consistently avoided gossip and watercooler stuff and only focused on the results that were needed," he says. "And that you pride yourself on that kind of professionalism."

Don't be a toady. Some people recommend that you emulate the boss—right down to wearing the same tasseled loafers and mimicking his speech patterns. The theory is that if you're like him, he will be more apt to feel comfortable with you and reward you. "Total garbage," Dr. Weiss says. "It's manipulative. It's dishonest and it's often transparent. You should dress professionally, but you have to be who you are. Nobody likes having toadies around."

Keep it strictly professional. Don't plead for a raise because others in your office got one. Nor should you cite the fact that you have a mortgage to pay and a family to feed, Dr. Weiss cautions. Others are in the same situation, and it's irrelevant, he says. "It should always be based on evidence."

If You Fail

Okay, you gave it your best shot, and the boss said no. After you finish sticking pins in the voodoo doll with his picture on it, consider these moves.

Be persistent. If the boss doesn't commit one way or another to your request, ask him what would be an appropriate follow-up or what you should do next, says Dr. Weiss. Don't let him get away with a comment such as, "Thanks, I'll get back to you."

Get a reason. If your request for a raise or a promotion is rejected, ask why. There could be a good reason, says Dr. Weiss. "If so, going to another job isn't going to help, because whatever it was that held you back would hold you back there."

Ask for perks. Even if your bid for more pay or a promotion is turned down, you can

---

You Should Play for the Milwaukee Bucks

Here's something to make you feel even worse the next time you get your annual 3 percent pay raise. Kevin Garnett, a forward with the NBA's Minnesota Timberwolves, saw his average salary jump 10-fold in one year. Garnett was making a paltry $2.1 million a season when he signed a six-year contract for $126 million—an average of $21 million per year.

So why can't you negotiate a similar deal for yourself where you work?

"The difference is that this guy might draw millions of dollars into the seats—the millions of dollars that result from championship or playoff games," says the Summit Consulting Group's Dr. Alan Weiss. "That's the return on investment."

Every time a company hires somebody from the outside, it's making an investment on return, too, because it doesn't know how the employee will perform. But when an insurance company hires an underwriter, the return is nowhere near the same as in professional sports, so the investment is much less.

"If you look at an athlete who has performed well, and he suddenly renegotiates his contract, the reason is that he has just demonstrated an outstanding couple of years and there is every reason to expect another outstanding couple of years," says Dr. Weiss. "It's the same thing in any organization. When somebody has a couple of fine years behind him, he's in a much stronger position to negotiate."

---

come out ahead, says Dr. Mercer. See if you can negotiate some job perks—the company paying your expenses to a convention or two, more vacation days, use of a company car or a car allowance, or use of a mobile phone, for example.

Give a Great Speech

At least one study has shown that people's number one fear in life is public speaking—it even ranks ahead of death. "To the average person, that means that if they have to go to a funeral, they'd be better off in the casket than giving the eulogy," comedian Jerry Seinfeld wrote in *SeinLanguage*.

The fear of dying in front of an audience—figuratively, if not literally—can give you cold sweats when you have to give a speech or make a presentation at work. Visions of your career flaming out faster than Brian Bosworth's dance in your head. Don't despair. Here are some things you can do to make that speech special.

The Art of the Spiel

Calm your nerves. One way to do so is to picture yourself giving your audience information that is valuable to them, says Spring Asher, co-owner of Chambers and Asher Speechworks, an Atlanta communications consulting firm. This takes your thoughts off yourself and puts the emphasis on the listeners, she says.

Grab their attention. "When you come into the room, your listeners look up and see you. You have 90 seconds to grab their attention at the beginning of a presentation," says Asher. "You don't want to waste it with 'Good afternoon, I'm glad to be here with you today.' You want to start out with a gee whiz fact or a story that relates to your subject."

And tell the audience why they will benefit from listening to what you are about to say, suggests Asher, who with partner Wicke Chambers wrote the book *Wooing and Win-*

ning Business. Then deliver on what you promise.

Say what you're going to say. Provide a sort of verbal table of contents by telling what three points you intend to make in your talk, in order to give listeners a road map of where you are going, Asher says.

Illustrate those points. Provide evidence to support your position. Do so by using anecdotes, statistics, personal examples, analogies, quotations, and experts' testimony or opinions, Asher says. "These are the things that bring your points to life."

Skip the jokes. There is no need to start a talk with humor, Asher says. "Speaking has changed," she says. "Young people don't want old-timey jokes. People want news they can use."

Look 'em in the eye. You don't need to memorize your entire speech, but you should know much of it without referring to notes, Asher says. "If you're going to read your presentation, you need to send a memo instead," she says. "The point of giving a presentation is to build a relationship and trust with your listener, and you can't do that if you're looking at a piece of paper." Eye contact is one of the two most important things in being an effective speaker, she adds.

Speak with enthusiasm. The other most important aspect of a good presentation is what Asher calls voice energy. No matter how scintillating your subject matter and how profound your knowledge of it, you will bore your audience if you use the same inflection that you did when you were a kid reciting the Gettysburg Address. "Sound like you have conviction," Asher suggests.

More than 90 percent of the reaction to your speech will be due to your physical presence and the tone of your voice, Asher says. The content counts for very little. But without a good knowledge of the content, you won't have the confidence to do those other things that make a good impression, she says.

Avoid using jargon. Using corporate buzzwords and phrases won't help you sell your ideas and may cost you some listeners, Asher says. "Keep it simple. Talk to the lowest common denominator. Then everybody is going to get it."

Pace yourself. In your desire to get the ordeal over with, you may hurry through your talk. Don't. Pause after each major point you make, Asher says. "Let the information sink in." At the same time, a brisk, albeit unhurried, speaking manner is effective, she adds. "People think you're smarter if you talk a little faster."

Practice good posture. Don't slouch. Stand on the balls of your feet. Begin the presentation with your hands at your sides, then gradually gesture toward your listeners. Don't assume a fig leaf posture or cross your arms. "The goal is to look open," Asher says. "Hands in your pockets is fine, but don't hold anything. It's a distraction."

Look around. Rather than standing stiffly at the podium throughout your talk, work the room a bit, Asher suggests. While you talk, make a visual connection with one person, then another and another. "When you have a large audience, everybody in the area in which you are looking thinks you're talking to him," she says.

Reaching the End Zone

Finishing strong is crucial to making a great speech. If you want your audience to walk out afterwards talking about what a dynamic speaker you are, keep the following tips in mind.

Recap. After you've discussed each of your points, it's important that you summarize

Maximum Mouth

Fidel Castro . . . now there's a public speaker. Cuba's "Maximum Leader" has given thousands of speeches, some running five hours or longer, with the record being around nine hours, according to author Tad Szulc, in his biography of Castro, *Fidel: A Critical Portrait*.

If you live in Cuba and watch television, you may be hard pressed to avoid a Castro soliloquy. Many of the bearded, camouflage-clad leader's talks are carried live on television—in their entirety—with several taped rebroadcasts over national channels, sometimes for a period of days. Castro's public appearances also are carried live in special reports or as part of the regular news programs, according to Szulc.

The hammy Castro reportedly claims to get stage fright before he launches into his loquacious musings. As a young man, he overcame this reticence by forcing himself to deliver speeches in front of a mirror in his room until he believed they were good enough that he could pursue a career in law and politics.

them. "You won't score if you don't bring it home," Asher says.

Tell them where to go. Yeah, we know: You'd *love* to tell them all where to go. But in this case, your speech should clearly answer the question of what action you want taken as a result of your message.

Don't bluff. If, when you finish, somebody asks you a question to which you don't know the answer, don't pretend you do know, Asher says. Admit that you don't know, and say that you'll get back to him with the answer. Or get your listeners involved by asking if anybody in the room knows the answer.

Run a Meeting

Before you schedule your next meeting, ask yourself this one simple question: Is this meeting really necessary?

"Meetings are a plague worthy of being minimized, and if you have to have them, make them count. Make them short and productive, and people won't hate going," says Eric Sundstrom, Ph.D., professor of psychology at the University of Tennessee in Knoxville and a consultant to businesses for more than two decades. Too many meetings are "talking bulletin boards" to give information that easily could have been disseminated by telephone or e-mail, he adds.

Realize also, however, that the ability to run productive, interesting meetings can make people who matter take notice of you. "It's really where leadership is seen," says Wicke Chambers, co-owner of Chambers and Asher Speechworks, an Atlanta communications consulting firm. "It's a wonderful career builder."

Remember rule one: Only schedule a meeting if there is a clear purpose that can best be accomplished by gathering people together in the same room. Provided that's the case, here's how to make every meeting minute count.

Have your own agenda. Prepare an agenda and distribute it in advance of the meeting, says Dr. Sundstrom. "You're asking someone to invest a certain amount of time for whatever purpose, so it would be nice to know ahead of time what the desired outcome is and what the agenda to get to that outcome is," he says.

A timed agenda in which a certain number of minutes are allocated for each item helps keep a meeting focused. Designate somebody to be the timekeeper, and agree on how he will signal that you are running long on a topic, advises Dr. Sundstrom.

Open strong. Immediately tell your listeners how the meeting will impact them, says Chambers. Make it clear at the outset why they should care about listening to you, whether the issue is job safety, productivity, or profits.

Try opening with a provocative question. Ask the group why companies buy—or don't buy—your products, for example. "Get people involved," says Chambers. "If you want people to come to your meeting and you want them to come on time, the fun stuff is up front. You want them to think, 'I don't want to miss the start of this meeting, because that's when the action is.'"

Stand tall. You don't necessarily need to stand up when you lead a meeting, but it can make listeners pay more attention, Chambers says. "I think standing is always much more commanding."

Keeping Things Moving

Getting their attention is only half the battle. Keeping it is the other half. Here's how to keep your meeting motoring along like a finely tuned Porsche.

Ask what they think. The meeting you run will be more interesting to your listeners if you involve them in the discussions, so ask for their feedback, Dr. Sundstrom suggests. But you don't want to make anybody feel like the kid in class who gets called on by the teacher and doesn't know the answer. So what do you do?

Ask questions of the group as a whole, but make eye contact with them individually, one at a time, says Dr. Sundstrom.

Break down. Another option is to break participants into small groups to discuss solutions or recommendations, Chambers says. This way, shy employees may feel more comfortable piping up, and one participant always emerges as the spokesperson for each group. That in itself is beneficial if you are a manager evaluating your personnel. "That says leadership and risk-taker."

Battle boredom. If your listeners are stifling more yawns than a convention of insomniacs, move on to the next agenda item, says Chambers. Keep the meeting moving briskly. "The point is not to be able to fulfill the mission, necessarily. It is to put people into action."

Take a break. If it's a very long meeting, schedule a break. "My experience is that if you don't have a break every 75 to 90 minutes, you better plan on people trickling in and out, and their minds wandering," says Dr. Sundstrom.

Be precise. Don't put words in the mouths of your listeners when summarizing points they have made, says Dr. Sundstrom. "Some people will correct you and others won't," he says. "They'll just be irritated later." To ensure accuracy if it's an important point, repeat back to participants what they just said and ask if you got it right.

Delegate responsibility. In addition to making one person responsible for keeping track of the time spent on agenda items, have somebody be in charge of recording comments and decisions made on a flip-chart if one is being used, says Dr. Sundstrom. This relieves you of the temptation to impose your own wording on the group's agreement and frees you to lead the meeting, instead of being the scribe.

Bite your tongue. If you have more authority than your listeners, give your opinion last or not at all, Dr. Sundstrom says. Nothing will dampen discussion faster than having the boss stake out a position first.

Take the next step. At the end of the meeting, recap and review what has been decided, recommends Chambers. Assign responsibilities and deadlines. Determine the follow-up process. "People want confirmation

---

Buzzword Bingo

You're making a salient point three-quarters of the way through the meeting you're leading when Farnsworth murmurs, "Bingo!" from the rear of the room. Everybody else smiles slightly and nods discreetly. Glad to see they all agree with me, you think to yourself.

In fact, your colleagues may simply be playing "Buzzword Bingo," a game devised for those who must endure endless meetings at which guys like you lapse into corporate jargon—also known as buzzwords.

So the next time you hear yourself saying that your company must be more proactive, that it must develop more synergy between departments and position itself for future challenges, beware that your colleagues could be counting every cliché.

It works like this. Employees compile their favorite corporate-culture clichés in bingo-card form. Then they surreptitiously take them into meetings and check off the buzzwords as the speaker intones them. First one to cover five squares in a row wins.

There even are Internet sites that provide made-to-order buzzword lists or allow Web surfers to print out Buzzword Bingo cards for free.

---

that they showed up, they contributed, and there is forward action." This is the time to give them that.

Evaluate the meeting. Either verbally or with a written form, ask participants to evaluate how well the meeting addressed the major points on the agenda, suggests Dr. Sundstrom. Then discuss it for a few minutes. If you conduct lots of meetings with the same people every time, do this only at the close of the first couple of such confabs. After that, it becomes less effective.

Fire Somebody

There was a time when it was relatively easy to move the dead wood out of your office. You simply said, "You're fired." A common-law concept called employment at-will made this possible. An employer could can a worker for any or no reason as long as no union or other contract was broken and discrimination laws weren't violated.

At-will is still around, but numerous state and federal laws and judicial rulings have made terminating an employee a lot dicier than it used to be, says attorney John C. Patzke, a partner in the Milwaukee law firm of Brigden and Petajan, which represents management in labor and employment matters.

Nowadays an employer can end up in court for terminating a worker in violation of numerous laws, including those governing people with disabilities, whistle-blowers, and sexual harassment. And in court is the last place you ever want to find yourself. So it helps to know the rules you're playing by these days.

From the first day that an employee walks in your door, there are steps you can take that will help you cover your assets and the company's. Here are a few of them.

Be honest. "Never promise anything you're not prepared to carry through with," Patzke cautions. Don't, for example, promise a new hire that his job will be safe for five years, then terminate him sooner because you want to save money.

Keep clear documents. Document what you expect of employees, along with their shortcomings and strengths, Patzke advises. "One of the pitfalls I always see is that nobody puts on a date," he says. "Or if they put a date, it's something like 6/26 and no year. Also, put your initials on documents you create."

Don't, however, keep documentation only on troublesome employees. "That leaves the impression you're out to get that person," Patzke says.

Evaluate accurately. Managers sometimes are tempted to give poor employees mediocre rather than bad annual job evaluations, Patzke says. That's because they fear that bad workers reflect negatively on themselves, and because it spares them the painful process of confronting workers about their shortcomings.

"It's going to come back and bite you in the shorts later, because eventually your bad employees will become so bad you're going to have to do something about them," Patzke says. Firing them later becomes problematic—how could these workers know they were remiss since their evaluations said otherwise? And how can you convince a jury that what you did was necessary?

Only fire as a last resort. "I've found it more profitable to try to turn the person around," says Beverly McHugh, owner of Business Services, a chain of professional employer organizations in Santa Clara, California. McHugh does this by offering the employee encouragement and trying to include him in the solution. "When I can get him to see it from my point of view, it is very effective," she says.

On the Firing Line

Before you fire or discipline an employee, be sure you can answer yes to each of the following questions, Patzke advises.

- Did the employee know the rule and the consequences of violating it?
- Is the rule reasonable?
- Did the employee disobey the rule?
- Was a fair investigation conducted?
- Is there proof that the employee is responsible for the behavior?
- Have the rules been consistently applied?
- Does the penalty match the offense?

If you answer yes to all of the above questions, it's time to act. Here's what you should do.

Give short notice. "You don't tell people two or three days in advance that you want to meet with them regarding their employment," Patzke says. "You don't want them to dwell on it and plot." Plot what? Punching you out—or worse.

Change your pattern. Similarly, if you make it a practice to always terminate workers at 4:00 P.M. on Fridays, the next guy you dismiss will figure out his fate when you tell him you want to speak alone with him at that time. Vary the times at which you take care of this unpleasant business.

Clear a path. Don't sit between the guy you're about to fire and the door. If he wants to flee the room, he should have easy access, Patzke says. And so should you.

Have a witness. When you do fire an employee, have a colleague with you as a witness. This can help later if there is a dispute over what was said, Patzke says. And the witness can give you a nudge if you're off base—for example, if you lose your temper.

Stick to business. In your guilt over firing somebody, don't tell him how great he is, Patzke advises. This gives him a mixed message and he may wonder, "If I'm so good, why are they firing me? Is there some other, secret reason?"

Elicit a response. Ask the worker you're terminating if there is any reason why you shouldn't do this. Give him his day in court if he cites his four kids or his huge mortgage payment. Listen politely, but don't be swayed, Patzke says. You're looking only for a reason that might be legally unfair. If there is one, tell him you will suspend rather than fire him until you investigate further.

"If you're ever in doubt about whether you should fire the person right then and there, don't do it," Patzke says. "Wait until you have the facts and you've given yourself enough time to reflect."

Watch him pack. Accompany the employee to his desk if he wants to remove his things right away, Patzke says. This way you can make sure he doesn't take confidential records or destroy computer files. Offer to arrange for somebody to meet him after hours to clean out his desk if he would prefer to do so without the stares of co-workers.

Going to Your Backhand

You canned that employee who charged a hooker to his expense account and now he has the brass to ask you for a letter of recommendation. You don't want to slander the hapless heel, nor do you wish to mislead future prospective employers.

The solution? Write a letter that tells it both ways. Robert Thornton, Ph.D., professor of economics at Lehigh University in Bethlehem, Pennsylvania, has made it easy in his book *Lexicon of Intentionally Ambiguous Recommendations.* Some examples:

Recommendation	Translation
"A man like him is hard to find."	He disappears frequently.
"He's a man of many convictions."	He has a record a mile long.
"He is definitely a man to watch."	I don't trust him.
"I wouldn't hesitate to give her an unqualified recommendation."	She just doesn't have the skills for the job.
"You will be very fortunate to get this person to work for you."	She's not very industrious.
"Waste no time in making this candidate an offer of employment."	She's not worth further consideration.

Cope with Being Fired

Not many people feel sorry for highly paid professional athletes when they lose their jobs, but jocks feel the same pain and confusion when they are cut that the rest of us do when we're given a pink slip. Just ask former NFL quarterback Jim Zorn.

Zorn was released in 1985 by the Seattle Seahawks after having been one of the team's premier players during most of his nine seasons there. Now it was as if none of that mattered.

"You have this feeling that all that you did wasn't very valuable," recalls Zorn, now the quarterbacks' coach for the Detroit Lions. "I had the feeling that I had failed. As I was driving out of the driveway when I got cut, the team was practicing. I was thinking they should stop practice for a week in remembrance of me."

Zorn's reaction was typical. Men generally take a job loss harder than women, says Ellie Wegener, executive director of the Employment Support Center in Washington, D.C., which provides assistance to the unemployed. "A man defines his job as the major thing in his life, and everything else is a little bit peripheral," she says.

No wonder that men are often devastated. "There is an immediate period of shock, just as there would be in any unexpected crisis," says Isabel Sodickson, a clinical social worker in Waban, Massachusetts. "Many people are actually quite surprised and unsettled to find that they are now having difficulty in many—or sometimes all—aspects of their lives."

Despite their feelings of failure, many people who are fired are victims of circumstances such as personality clashes or company changes that have nothing to do with their competence. "Unfortunately, bad things do happen to good people," says Sodickson.

Another former NFL quarterback, Babe Parilli, knows this well. He quarterbacked coaching legend Vince Lombardi to his first win with the Green Bay Packers. His reward? "He cut me," recalls Parilli, who then played another decade in the pros.

What to Do First

As soon as you're terminated, determine whether you qualify for unemployment benefits. If you do, file a claim at your local unemployment office. This will partially offset the loss of income you are about to experience, Wegener says.

Now, it's time to get on with the rest of your life. Here are some steps to help make the transition easier.

Join the club. By joining a support group or job club, a guy meets other competent men who also are out of work, Wegener says. It's helpful for guys to swap work-related stories and offer encouragement to one another, she says. This also prevents men from isolating themselves from others, which is the worst thing they can do right now.

Support groups usually work best when professionals are all in one and blue-collar workers are grouped in another, Wegener says. "The pain is the same, but the way that you look at your job and try to find another job is quite different. Having buddies around makes you feel better."

It's important to talk to somebody about your firing in order for you to move on, Wegener adds. "If you can get it out of your system, that will help you a lot."

Keep the faith. Belief in a higher power helps get you through a crisis like losing your job, says ex-quarterback Zorn. "Had I not been a Christian and believed that God is in control of my circumstances, then I think I would have had a much rougher time," he says. "I knew my life wasn't over."

Take a trip. If you've lost your job, chances are you can't afford a vacation unless you got a handsome severance package or saved wisely. But consider getting away for a few days, even if you just go back-packing, Wegener suggests. "Use the time to renew your energy, your mind, your whole self, but *don't* think about how horrible life is."

Start looking. Even if you get away for a few days, don't wait too long to start looking for another job, Wegener advises. "The less time spent on the negative and agonizing over it, the better," she says. "The people who work at it hardest and most intelligently are the people who get the jobs."

Become a volunteer. It's a way to keep busy and feel useful while you're out of work, Wegener says. Or get involved in self-improvement activities such as an exercise program or a new interest, Sodickson adds. This can give your self-esteem a needed boost. "The general thinking is that success in some areas of life can contribute to success in other areas," Sodickson says.

The Last Laugh

Getting fired can be a good move. Take a look at the jobs some celebrities held before they found their calling.

Celebrity	Former Job
Marlon Brando	Department store elevator operator
Gene Hackman	Ladies' shoe salesman at Saks in New York
Steve Martin	Sold Mouseketeer ears and Davy Crockett coonskin hats at Disneyland
Brad Pitt	Wore a giant chicken suit outside a fast-food restaurant
Frank Zappa	Greeting card designer and encyclopedia salesman
Sean Connery	Milkman and coffin polisher
Rod Stewart	Grave digger
Joe Cocker	Plumber
Chuck Berry	Hairdresser
Lawrence Welk	Farmer

Finding Another Job

Think about what you want to do with the rest of your working life, Wegener advises. "If you hated the job you were fired from—which is sometimes why people were fired—then for heaven's sake, don't try to get the same job," she says.

Changing careers can be daunting. You may feel that whatever your last job was is all that you are trained for, all that you know. Ask a job counseling service if they have a personality or aptitude test you can take to determine where your other talents may lie.

Here are some additional things you can do.

Network. Get over any embarrassment you may have about being unemployed and contact as many friends and acquaintances as you can and ask them if they know of job opportunities, Wegener suggests. Even if they don't work in the same field as you, they may be able to recommend a friend of a friend in your line of work.

Get a letter. Seek a letter of recommendation or a reference from the job where you were fired, especially if you worked there for any length of time, Wegener says. The person who actually canned you may be unable or unwilling to provide such a letter, but somebody else with the company—even a higher-ranking manager—may do so.

Be positive. Tell prospective new employers as little as possible about your firing, Wegener suggests. Simply say you had a difference of opinion over how to run the company or do the job. Don't bad-mouth the person who fired you—whoever is interviewing you will wonder if they are in for the same treatment if they hire you.

"You should certainly not hide the fact that you were fired, because it's too easy to find out," Wegener adds. The only exception is a job you were at so briefly that you opt not to include it on your résumé.

Get a Leave of Absence

Going to the office has become as much fun as a stroll to the electric chair? You'd like to take six months off so you can finally surf the Banzai Pipeline? Or maybe you'd simply like a respite from work so you can carefully catalog and review all of your back issues of *Men's Health*. Regardless of the reason, seeking a leave of absence is risky business. The rules of disengagement are best negotiated with a guide. One follows.

When to Seek a Leave

First, be forewarned: The climate in today's leaner, meaner working world is hardly conducive to following your dreams.

"Taking a leave of absence is going to shoot a hole in your boat in terms of your career," warns industrial psychologist Dr. Michael Mercer. "The only way to justify a long leave of absence is to have a compelling reason that means you cannot be at work." Among those reasons:

- Parental leave because of the birth of a child
- Family illness that requires you to leave the area
- Educational experience such as a fellowship at a university in a field of study that is related to your job, or another educational program that is reimbursed by your company
- Community service such as working for a nonprofit agency
- Running for office, or helping your spouse do so

"All of these reasons are developing a person, presumably keeping him personally and professionally healthier when he returns to work," says the Summit Consulting Group's Dr. Alan Weiss. "But if you just want to go and lose yourself in the world for a year, you're entitled to do that, but there is no reason the company should safeguard your job while you do it."

By Your Leave

You've figured out what you want to do. Now you need to figure out how to get your company to let you do it. Here's how.

Be realistic. "If you're a production worker at a plastics manufacturer, the chances of getting a sabbatical to study hieroglyphics in Egypt are going to be pretty low," says attorney Jim Kuns, a staff consultant at the Employers Group, a Los Angeles company that has provided human resources management services for more than 100 years. "If you're in a more professional position like that of a professor, they would be higher."

Increase your odds. Working extra hard to carve a specialized niche for yourself in the company is a great trump card to play when the time comes to ask for a leave. "The more valuable you are, the more the company will bend over backward for you," says Dr. Mercer. "If it's hard to replace you and you say you absolutely need to do this, your chances are better."

Consider your benefits. If you take an unpaid leave of absence, you're not only forgoing your income but also probably your benefits. "The basic rule of thumb is that if you're going out on a nonpaid status, the company is most likely not going to let you accrue vacation time or sick leave," Kuns says. So calculate what the real cost will be, and then decide if you can afford it.

Ask your boss first. If you go initially to your company's human resources office seeking a leave of absence, "you come off like some namby pamby nit-picking jerk" quoting company policy, says Dr. Mercer. You don't work for human resources, you work for your boss, so go to him first. If he really needs you on his team, he can—perhaps reluctantly—expedite your request.

"If the only reason you can take a leave of absence is because of a policy, your boss will want to fire you," says Dr. Mercer. That's because he may perceive you as unconcerned with his department's performance and trying to circumvent him by making your request to another department.

Get it in writing. If you are approved for a leave of absence, insist on having the terms in writing, says Dr. Weiss. Such a document might include the length of time you will be gone along with language stipulating that when you return to work, you will get your job or an equivalent position. Do this even if you trust your boss and your company.

"I always work on the beer truck principle," says Dr. Weiss. "That is, what if the person who guaranteed you this gets hit by a beer truck? You have to have it in writing. The company could be purchased. All sorts of things could happen."

Get more than one approval. At the very least, get a senior manager and the vice president of human resources to sign off on your leave of absence, advises Dr. Weiss. "It's always best having as many signatures as you can. That way you're doubly safe."

Lay Down the Law

Depending on your job and your circumstances, a leave of absence needn't always be at the discretion of your boss. You may have the law on your side. The federal Family and Medical Leave Act of 1993 entitles

Family Ties

When Rick Seid took a three-month sabbatical in 1997, he did something some men never make time for. The self-professed workaholic got to know his family better.

Director of human resource services and systems at Watson Wyatt Worldwide in Bethesda, Maryland, Seid bicycled through England with his 13-year-old son, took his entire family—he also has a daughter—to the North Carolina coast for 3 weeks, visited his parents in Las Vegas, and spent 2½ weeks in Bermuda with his wife.

Of the bicycling trip with son Matt, Seid says: "I learned he is grown-up and independent, and he has a mind of his own. He's doing pretty good on the maturity side—I was surprised."

He also is grateful that the sabbatical enabled him to see his father, who died shortly after Seid returned to work. "We had some good conversations," he recalls. "We finally got to know each other after quite a few years."

Seid helped create his company's policy on sabbaticals and was one of the initial group of 11 workers to use it. Watson Wyatt, which is a consultant on human resource issues, makes high-performing employees eligible for a sabbatical after 10 years. The company allows sabbaticals of up to three months and pays two-thirds of the worker's salary.

"The bottom line is that the company and our clients are benefiting from having these persons re-energize themselves," Seid says.

eligible employees to take as much as 12 weeks of unpaid, job-protected leave in a 12-month period for specified family and medical reasons.

Join the Circus

Who among us hasn't considered packing it in for life under the big top? The camaraderie and intrigue from living among a nomadic community of performers.... The buzz of excitement rippling through the crowds.... The babes in the circus and in every audience gazing adoringly as you... you... do what?

Hmmm. Your college didn't offer a course in Trapeze 101. Your dad never taught you how to juggle. You've been called a clown, but you lack formal training. What do you do?

Well, it depends on the type of job.

Chances are, if you've been holding down a regular 9-to-5 job, you haven't been honing your skills on the high wire or as an elephant trainer. That being the case, you won't land a circus job with the greatest of ease. Here's what you can do to better your chances.

Go to school. Enroll at a school that teaches various circus skills. Among the possibilities: the San Francisco School of Circus Arts; Lebrecque Studios Performing Arts Center in Lynbrook, New York; and Dell' Arte School of Physical Theatre in Blue Lake, California, which isn't technically a circus school, but includes instruction in circus arts such as acrobatics and juggling, in addition to work in clown, mime, and other physical comedy.

Or you might enroll at Florida State University in Tallahassee to learn circus skills and perhaps perform with the school's talented Flying High Circus. Triton College in River Grove, Illinois, also has a circus class and performers. In Canada, you could train at the National Circus School in Montreal.

Make a video. Once you've developed some talents, make a video and send it and a résumé out to some of the circuses. "Quite often, we'll have people come out and audition for the show. They can do a split and a somersault, but that's no circus act. You have to be able to put together a complete act with four or five major tricks, plus have some wardrobe, a nice appearance, and some style about you," says Ted Bowman, who was an executive with Carson and Barnes Circus, based in Hugo, Oklahoma. For 31 years, Bowman worked for the circus, doing everything from bookkeeping, publicity, and serving as show manager and equestrian director, to having his own elephant act.

Marry into the life. "We have a lot of performing families in our show that are third and fourth generation," says Alfrieda Wilkins, another Carson and Barnes official. Sometimes, novices marry into circus performing families and eventually learn to perform with them, she says.

Indeed, Carson and Barnes often hires "by the family," Bowman says. Not everybody in the group will necessarily be a family member, but the group will be offered a flat rate—perhaps $2,500 to $3,500 a week—depending on how many acts they perform, he explains. Somebody in the "family" must then determine how to divvy up the dough among members.

About two-thirds of circus jobs aren't those of glamorous performers but of support people. Pay is much lower, turnover is much higher. Most jobs provide communal meals. Some also provide transportation and sleeping quarters—a bus, truck, or trailer. You may land one of these jobs by simply contacting a circus when it comes to your town or writing to the outfit. Among the jobs:

- Electricians
- Truck drivers ("We are always needing drivers," Wilkins says.)
- Mechanics
- Concession operators
- "Care-fors"—guys who care for animals, shoveling their poop and feeding and washing them
- Guys to "run canvas"—that is, erect and take down the big top in every town

A guy who is a reliable worker in one of these jobs might advance to a job inside the tent, says Wilkins. Somebody whose job is to put up and take down the big top may move inside to run a concession, for example. Or a guy following the elephants around with a shovel could move up to performing with some of the animals if he is good with them.

The Life

The life of a circus performer may be harder than you imagine. At Carson and Barnes, the season runs from March through November. During those months, the entourage is performing and traveling seven days a week. In 1997, this five-ring circus visited 136 cities and towns in the western United States.

Most circuses don't usually play before the bright lights of New York City and Las Vegas. They are more apt to pull into towns such as La Porte, Indiana, and Coppell, Texas.

"We like to play towns of around 20,000 people," says Wilkins. "It's hard work, in all kinds of weather, in all locations. Sometimes, we're digging our way out of mud. Sometimes, we're coping with dust storms."

Most circus people don't get rich. Performers make the most money by far—$500 to $2,000 a week plus meals is the range at Carson and Barnes, Wilkins says.

During the season, many performers travel in expensive recreational vehicles and motor homes, and they often own homes that they return to in the off-season, says Trey Key, a general agent with Kelly-Miller Circus, based in Hugo, Oklahoma. But laborers may make only $150 to $200 a week, plus meals, a bunk, and perhaps transportation.

Says Bowman, "It's a hard life. It's a business you absolutely have to love or you're going to hate it."

The Graduate

It's doubtful that this is what Trey Key's parents had in mind when they sent him off to school at prestigious Brown University in Providence, Rhode Island, where tuition tops $20,000 a year. After graduating in 1989 with a degree in ethics and political philosophy, Key promptly enrolled in another school—the Ringling Brothers Clown College. He graduated again and joined the Kelly-Miller Circus. After one season of clowning, this Ivy League grad took a succession of other jobs—press agent, booking agent, and now general agent, supervising the press and booking agents.

Circus life can be a grind, but the glamour is real—at least for the performers, Key says. "The payoff is the performance," says Key. "It's when people applaud and the performers' families and friends get to come and see them."

In case you're wondering—and we know that you are—circuses do have the equivalent of groupies, says Key. There usually are a few girls who are gaga over the "flying boys" and other performers and who hang around after shows, he says. But smaller circuses are on the move so quickly that it's hard to find time for romance on the road, he adds.

Still, Key likes the life. "I always considered being out on the road as a press agent as kind of an eight-month vacation—just never let your boss know how much fun your job is."

Be a Hobo

A hobo's life is happy,
a hobo's life is free,
It's a life of travelin' all around,
and that's the life for me.
I'm just a guy that won't fit in,
I've always been that way.
I'm catchin' out for freedom,
I'm leavin' today.
—Guitar Whitey, *Catchin' Out for Freedom*

Sitting in our cars at a railroad crossing watching a train rumble past, it can seem mighty tempting to join Guitar Whitey. Leave behind debts and deadlines for a life ridin' the rails. Feel the wind in our hair as we peer out of a boxcar at a lonesome prairie. Oh, and adopt a cool moniker like Fry Pan Jack or Oklahoma Slim.

Just what constitutes a hobo, however, is subject to debate. "A hobo is someone who rides freight trains to find work and to travel," says Marie Steenlege, former director of the chamber of commerce in Britt, Iowa, home of the National Hobo Convention, which is held every year. "They were wandering workers."

Purists would agree. Controversies have arisen over the choosing of a king of the hoboes every year, because some of those anointed have been regarded as mere recreational train-hoppers, Steenlege says.

Today's hoboes "are nothing but would-be hoboes and rubber-tire hoboes" or hitchhikers, says Rambling Rudy of Shawneetown, Illinois, a hobo from 1925 to 1932 who was named hobo of the year in 1986.

Old-timers like Rambling Rudy cadged many a free meal by knocking on a stranger's back door, hat in hand. They ranked meals the following way, he says.

Set-down. "You go in the house and set down with the family."

Knee-shaker. "They put a plate of food on you, you put it on your lap, set at the back door, and try to eat it while the chickens and dog try to eat at the same time."

Leper handout. "They hand it to you and you're told to move on."

Can a hobo still manage this way? "You couldn't do it today," says Rambling Rudy. "Today you go to a back door, they'll shoot you going across the yard. We always have the Salvation Army as a last resort. But it seemed like people had a kind heart for the hoboes back in the old days."

Oats, the hobo handle of a philosophy professor at an Illinois college, estimates that there are 150 to 250 full-time hoboes still riding the rails, and many more part-timers who travel only in warmer months.

Oats, who prefers that his real name and college affiliation not be used for this chapter, has attended hobo conventions and befriended hoboes. He also has compiled two books of poems written by hoboes and has ridden the rails on short journeys himself.

"They're a nice community," he says. "Friendly people. I like them."

Spiritual Quests, Kings and Queens

A philosophy professor in his fifties hardly seems the sort to hop freight trains and pal around with hoboes. "There's just something about being alone on that train, especially when you're out in the middle of Iowa, you can see the stars and nobody knows where you're at," Oats explains. "It's you, the train, God, and the stars. It's kind of like a spiritual quest."

In Britt, Iowa, it's also something of a fun quest. Every August about 50 hoboes and 20,000 other folks convene in the town of 2,100 for the hobo convention. Festivities include hoboes playing music and telling tales around a campfire at their camp, or "jungle," near the railroad tracks, and the naming of a king and queen of the hoboes.

There also is a parade down Main Street (the hoboes adorn one of the floats), a big outdoor flea market, the Hobo Run 5-K and 10-K races, and the serving of 500 gallons of Mulligan stew. On a more somber note, there is a memorial service for the hoboes buried in a specially designated area of Britt's cemetery. The town also has a hobo museum and a gift shop.

But while the thought of catchin' out for freedom is enticing, the truth is that hobo life is hard, says Oats, who does not recommend guys try it. "It's loneliness, cold, insecurity. It's illegal and dangerous. There are accidents. You can get killed."

If you were to become a hobo, however, here are some things to keep in mind.

Make sure you have what it takes. "You got to listen to that train whistle and you got to feel it," says Oats. "Without that passion, it's not going to be hoboing, it's just going to be a vacation."

Be self-sufficient. If you can't make it on your own, you can't make it as a hobo. Hoboes sometimes pair up and sometimes travel alone. Either way, your circle of friends is limited. "You need to be comfortable with yourself," says Oats.

Be willing to work. A hobo Oats knows named The Texas Madman sometimes supports his travels by picking crops. Others will stay in a town long enough to collect and sell aluminum cans for recycling. During the Depression, Rambling Rudy occasionally worked as a "pearl diver"—washing dishes and peeling potatoes in a café somewhere.

Don't drink and ride. Oats once met a fellow train rider whose buddy had just toppled

off a moving grain car—presumably to his death. The two had been drinking, he says.

Stop and go. Never get on or off a moving train, advises Oats. Modern trains accelerate very quickly, he adds.

Phone home. If you're in a relationship, let her know where you are. "I always call my wife whenever I get where I am," says Oats. "As soon as I get home, I call her at work."

Rambling Rudy Remembers

Rambling Rudy is reminiscing about the train he hopped to Tucson in 1928 because a restaurant there gave free food to hoboes.

"There was a hog trough behind that restaurant. About 100 of us hoboes lined up on each side and several times a day, two boys would come out and dump 10 gallons of garbage in it. As it went floating by, we'd grab it and throw it in our mouths. We hadn't eaten in two or three days, and we was hungry. Of course, after a handful or two of it, I told my buddy Hard Luck Slim, 'I think we can do better than this in Phoenix.'"

In Phoenix, the hoboes loitered outside a Catholic school until four nuns carried out tubs of oatmeal and the men dug in, eating with their hands. "It was good oatmeal," Rambling Rudy recalls. "I'm a missionary Baptist, but I learned early in life if you was hungry, you go to a Catholic school or a Catholic hospital or church and they never turn you down."

After seven years of the hobo life, Rambling Rudy, then 21, went to work at his father's lunch counter and spent the next 55 years in the restaurant business.

"Today I'm a pauper living on $400 a month Social Security," he says. "Money never did mean nothing to me. I've lived. I've got no complaints."

Become a Cowboy

If your idea of what cowboys are like comes from the movies and TV, you have the wrong idea, bucko. It's not all ridin' and ropin' and joining posses to pursue bad guys and tossing back shots in a saloon as you regale fellow cowpokes and the local floozies with tales of your heroic exploits.

"The misconception is that a cowboy is a hard-riding, hard-drinking, two-gun, two-fisted fclla," says Red Steagall, a cowboy, singer, and radio show host whom the Texas state legislature proclaimed the "Official Cowboy Poet of Texas."

"The truth is they are hard-working, honest, God-loving people who are really dedicated to their families," Steagall says.

So, pardner, you still want to be a cowboy? Let's see if you have what it takes.

The Job Description

So, what skills do you need on your résumé to land a job as a cowpoke? Read on.

Horsemanship. "That's not just being able to stay on a horse," Steagall says. "You need to understand something about training the animal."

Understanding livestock. "You have to be able to read cows," Steagall says. "In other words, you pretty much know what those cows are going to do before they do it."

Handling a rope. You must be able to rope cattle so you can move them from one area to another, brand them, and medicate them, says Tom Nall, owner of the Conejos Ranch in southern Colorado.

Branding. Cattle-rustling remains a problem out West, so ranchers brand their animals to identify them, Steagall says.

Castrating. Bulls need to be castrated so that they become more interested in eating than frolicking. "You take his mind off ass and put it on grass," Nall says. The result is a steer that is less muscular and produces tastier meat.

Veterinary care. A cowboy has to know how to administer vaccinations to cattle to protect them from disease. He may even have to serve occasionally as a bovine midwife. "If you have a calf not coming out right, you have to help," Steagall says.

Handy with tools. When he's not working with cattle, a cowboy may spend considerable time mending or building fences, says Nall.

The Cowboy Life

Don't look to strike it rich working as a cowboy. "It doesn't pay enough to be called an occupation—it's a way of life," Steagall says.

"It's having a trade just like a plumber, a welder, or a carpenter," Nall says. "But there's one major difference that makes it so romantic to me and I think most cowboys—you do your work on horseback."

A day-working cowboy works seasonally, traveling from one ranch to another. He makes about $55 to $60 a day, plus room and board, which is a bunkhouse or—less often—a bedroll by a chuck wagon that travels to the men in the pastures.

Large ranches, however, may have cowboys working exclusively for them. Single men typically sleep in a bunkhouse, while married cowboys live at camps. The latter often consist of a house, barn, horse corral, and working pens on the ranch owner's property. A huge ranch may have several camps, with each cowboy living there being responsible for a certain number of acres and head of cattle, Steagall says. The pay is about $1,200 a month, plus use of the house, a pickup truck, and one steer to slaughter for the cowboy's personal consumption.

Getting Hired

If you work a job where your heaviest exertion is opening the mail, breaking into the ranks of cowboys will be tougher than bad beef jerky. Most cowboys grew up on ranches, learning the skills and the lifestyle as kids, Steagall says. Still, there are a few things you can do.

Start at the bottom. You might gain experience by caring for animals at a dude ranch, then work your way up to other jobs so that you gain some further experience, Nall suggests. Or learn to be a farrier—that's someone who shoes horses, to you city slickers—or a cook to wrangle your way onto a ranch, then master other tasks once you've done so.

Go on cattle drives. Steagall and Nall are among those who take urban cowboys out on week-long cattle drives, like the one depicted in the comedy hit *City Slickers*, starring Billy Crystal and Jack Palance. The greenhorns help round up cattle from horseback and sleep on the ground near a chuck wagon every night.

The white-collar workers paying for the privilege learn bona fide cowboy skills. "Some of those guys who have been going for four or five years have actually become pretty good hands," Steagall says.

Go to college. You won't learn how to lasso a steer, but a lot of cowboys these days have college degrees in animal husbandry, Steagall says. And at least two universities offer range management courses. "If you had a degree in animal science and a certificate from a range management school, somebody would give you a chance," Steagall says. "You would understand the technical aspects of the lifestyle, and then you would have an opportunity to learn those basic skills."

Hey, Dude

Maybe the notion of castrating bulls, delivering calves, and riding the range in a thunderstorm has dampened your cowboy ardor. Still, the dream dies hard as a sun-baked prairie muffin. So consider a dude ranch.

There are more than 300 dude ranches in the West, says Jim Futterer, co-executive director of the Dude Ranchers' Association in Colorado. Some are working cattle ranches at which guests can help with a roundup, but most offer scenic horseback rides, cookouts, hayrides, and the like, Futterer says.

"You can go from rugged cowboy experiences to being fairly pampered," he says.

Guests typically stay at a dude ranch about a week, paying $1,100 to $1,200 a week per adult based on double occupancy, Futterer says. The price includes lodging, meals, and most activities except for such off-ranch outings as white-water rafting that may be arranged through a contractor.

If you're planning a stay at a dude ranch for the first time, Futterer suggests that you contact a state dude ranch association or write to his organization at Box 471, Laporte, CO 80535, for a free directory of more than 100 reputable dude ranches.

Practice. Steagall recalls working on a ranch where a young, untrained Swede came to work. "He would stand for hours just learning to swing a rope over his head before he ever threw it at anything," Steagall says. "If he wanted to learn to saddle a horse, he'd saddle that horse 100 times until he learned how tight to pull the cinch, how to put a bit in his mouth. When he left Texas and went back to Sweden, he was an outstanding cowboy."

Become a Swimsuit Photographer

We wanted to know: Is taking pictures of buxom babes in little-bitty bikinis as glamorous as it appears? "The worst day on the beach shooting bikini-clad women is better than the very best day on the assembly line," says Cliff Hollenbeck, a Seattle travel photographer, film producer, and author of numerous photography books, including *Swimsuit Model Photography*. "Even though it's work, it's probably the most fun you can have working."

And does that fun include being amorous with the models? Probably not.

"It's like watching a porno movie," Hollenbeck says. "The first five minutes are pretty interesting. After a while, it's a little bit boring. I'm thinking about the light, can I sell this. She's thinking about the same things."

There is no one path to follow to become a swimsuit photographer. Tom Mayes, a professional photographer in Oakland, California, got a business degree in college, took a single black-and-white photography darkroom course, and began teaching himself to become a photographer. Here are some things you might try.

Learn what you're doing. Read books, trade magazines, and photo supply catalogs to learn what equipment you need, lighting techniques, and the like, Hollenbeck says. Take a college course or attend seminars by professional shutterbugs.

Become a photo assistant. Take a job helping a successful photographer, suggests Mayes. You learn a lot about the business—from lighting to posing models to the financial end of things. "There are a lot of photo assistants who turn into great photographers," he says.

Get a girl. Hire a model from a modeling agency and practice the craft, says Hollenbeck. It may cost you from $50 an hour to $2,000 a day. Or go to a modeling school and hire an aspiring model for less money and give her some pictures for her portfolio in return.

Selling Your Pictures

Fashion companies, travel organizations, photo agencies, the Internet, and magazines are but a few of the markets for bikini photos. Still, making a sale is not easy.

"Just like a lot of women want to be models, a lot of guys want to be swimwear photographers simply because you get to deal with a lot of good-looking women," says Mayes. That means there's a glut of bikini images flooding the market, making it harder to make sales. If you insist on trying, though, follow these tips.

Be creative. "It entails more than a girl standing there," says Hollenbeck. "Get her in the surf and let the water jump up around her. Get her running with a beach ball. Put a set of fins in her hand. Make her come alive. I call that making a picture with impact."

Develop a portfolio. "Portfolios should be sweet and simple," says Hollenbeck. "Put your 10 best shots in it."

A portfolio is essential for face-to-face meetings with a prospective employer, says Mayes. But if you are marketing yourself by mail, make up something called zed cards. These postcardlike tools should feature 2 to 10 of your best images and information on how to contact you.

Sell yourself. Mayes once pestered the publisher of a bikini catalog for two years before convincing her to let him shoot pictures. "If you do a good job and market yourself a little bit, keeping yourself in front of people you want to be hired by, nothing beats that," he says.

Part Six

The Woman's Man

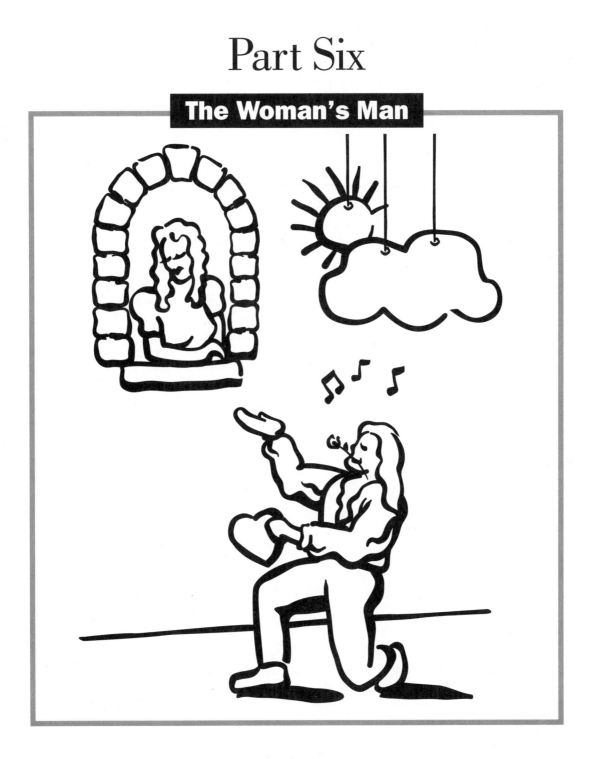

Get Back in the Game

It's been a while. Flustered, timid, tongue-tied, and unsure sum up how you're feeling. And you haven't even talked to a woman yet.

If eight-track tapes were the hottest thing on the market the last time you were on a date, this chapter's for you. But take heart—you're not alone. About half of us get another go at being single, thrown back into the whirling waters of unwed women. Consider this an opportunity to get it right.

The first thing you should know is that women's attitudes toward men with a courtly eye have changed. Today's women have heard it all before, says Lila Gruzen, Ph.D., a Sherman Oaks, California, relationship, marriage, and family therapist and coauthor of *Ten Foolish Dating Mistakes*. They're more worldly, more egalitarian, and less inclined to be forgiving of a man with awkward overtures.

That said, the basic emotional plumbing of women (and men, for that matter) remains the same, untouched by shades of Gloria Steinem. "Men and women are more alike than different," Dr. Gruzen says. "We all want the same things." That includes love, respect, a bite of the kids' Happy Meal, and, yes, even sex.

The New Rules

Gone are the days when you sidled up to a woman at a club, gave her an ogling look from Birkenstocks to beret, and invited her to come inspect the shag in your van.

"I know of so many women who say, 'I just wish he'd move his eyes up 10 inches,'" says Wendy Maltz, a certified sex therapist and counselor in Eugene, Oregon, and author of *Passionate Hearts: The Poetry of Sexual Love*.

So here a few important pointers to get you back into the swing of things.

Be light of heart. A sense of humor is often the most underused item in a man's chest of wooing tools, says Dr. Gruzen. "When men lose their sense of humor, it's a really fatal foolish dating mistake," she says. Women truly appreciate a man who can laugh and not take himself too seriously. How else can a short, fuzzy-headed guy like Billy Crystal get to hang out with Meg Ryan and Debra Winger?

Keep first dates short. In the initial stages, meeting for a cup of coffee is a great way to avoid investing too much time with someone who just isn't going to work out, says Dr. Gruzen. "If you go on long dinner dates and you end up hating the person sitting across from you, you get turned off to dating altogether," she says.

Don't give too much too soon. This can be money, gifts, information, whatever. People have a tendency to want to skip over the creepy, awkward stages of getting to know someone and develop intimacy as quickly as possible. "If you skip over that part, then you don't get to know them," Dr. Gruzen says. "You just get to know the fantasy, who you think they are."

Dodge the bullet. If in the initial stages of dating, she asks you to tell her about your ex, Dr. Gruzen has one emphatic word of advice—don't. "It's a trick question. If you hate her, you're not over her. If you like her, you're not over her either," she warns. Say something vague, like it just didn't work out, and move on.

Forget that she's a woman. Well, at least once you've established that she *is* a woman. "Put blinders on. Block out the person's genitals, their sexuality, and listen to what they have to say," Maltz suggests. You want to find out her hopes, her dreams, her beliefs. Let her tell you. Funny thing is, the best conversationalists are those who are the best listeners, Maltz says. "You can be aware of your sexual attraction, but just enjoy it on your own for a while." The best part is that she'll love you for it. After years of fending off crude sexual advances, she'll find you to be a breath of welcome spring air. And you know what happens in spring. . . .

Postpone the sex. Yeah, right, you say. We're serious here. It's not a moral or physical thing, although the specter of AIDS should have you thinking carefully before you hop in any bed. "Sex allows you to fall asleep for about a year in a relationship, and then you wake up and realize you know nothing about this person," Dr. Gruzen says. The bedroom can mask the fact that you're largely incompatible in every other way. And by the time you realize she's definitely not the one for you, she is wearing your clothes, has joined your health club, and is playing cards with your sister-in-law. It gets messy.

So, how long should you wait? "It's psychologically not in a man's best interest to have sex until at least three to four months into the relationship," says Dr. Gruzen. You'll know by then if you want to give her some space in your sock drawer.

Fix her an old-fashioned. If your last dates were, say, 15 to 20 years ago, you probably know some things that younger men find totally foreign. "I firmly believe that the old-fashioned manners, grace, and charm have never gone out of style," says Susan G. Rabin, a New York City relationship therapist, director of The School of Flirting, and author of *101 Ways to Flirt*. "Women still very much appreciate that." Younger men, she adds, have few of the social skills that their older counterparts have. Use that to your advantage. And as for that modern dilemma: "Picking up the check is never a turnoff to a woman," she says. There you have it.

Stranger Than Fiction

There are a lot of men out there with the pattern of a barroom floor imprinted squarely across their faces. This comes from falling flat on them after delivering a hopelessly bad pickup line.

While writing his book *How to "Pick Up" Beautiful Women*, former bartender John Eagan interviewed more than 2,000 women whom he considered beautiful, trying to discover what they look for in a man they are meeting for the first time. One of the questions he asked each woman was, What was the nicest, most unusual, or funniest line a man ever said to you? Here are some of the answers.

- "Wow! Great job, God."
- "My Jaguar needs an oil change. You want it?"
- "You remind me of my mother."
- "I would take you out for dinner, but I don't have any money."
- "Well, now you've done it. I'll have to dismiss my whole harem now that I met you."
- "I wish I had a higher IQ so I could enjoy your company."
- "Four out of five voices in my head recommended I come over and talk to you."
- "Would you mind talking to me now, because by the time I finish this drink, I'll be a slobbering idiot."
- "I'd take my pants off over my head for you."

You've heard a lot here about patience and taking it slow. For a reason. As in sex, women take longer to warm up to a relationship, says Maltz. But once they do, look out. "Men would score a lot more if they just learned the art of patience," she says. "Once a woman feels safe, she's pretty open. She's going to start moving on you."

Flirt with Flair

In the sometimes-barren landscape of workplace drudgery, crowded bars, and frenetic gyms, the smile from a comely female often breathes life back into a gray day. No wonder we flirt with them.

And though it may lead to a relationship, that's not always the aim. "No matter how happily a woman may be married," wrote the eminent U.S. journalist H. L. Mencken, "it always pleases her to discover that there is a nice man who wishes that she were not."

In order to flirt well, it's essential to know exactly what flirting is. "It's a charming and honest expression of interest in others," says Susan G. Rabin, a relationship therapist and the director of The School of Flirting. "Good flirts pay attention to other people; they make other people feel important and appreciated. It's a wonderful art."

Take note—it does not mean getting that head-turner down in purchasing alone in the file room. Nor does it mean sidling up to Sally Sloegin in a bar and trying to convince her to inspect the back seat of your Buick. "You can have sex on your mind, but keep it off your lips," Rabin says. "Women are so used to being sex objects and touched and pawed and called at. They're tired of that."

Is She Interested?

Consider flirting a form of social badminton. It takes two active participants, both volleying and returning. Without a willing partner, you may as well fire your birdie into the wall. So, the first thing you need to consider is whether she's up to a bit of court time with you. If she's not, back off and respect that decision.

Check for a green light. It's not too difficult to determine if a woman is interested in flirting with you, says Rabin. The problems begin when a man doesn't bother to stop and see. Uninvited advances are not flirtation, she stresses. Not only does that show poor taste on the part of the man but it may also constitute sexual harassment.

Pay attention. Look for telltale signs like a ready smile when she sees you approaching, suggests Rabin. If she buries her head in a file folder, it's best to move on. You may also notice her giving you short, sidelong glances during the course of the day. Another good sign. And she may actively seek you out for a chance to chat over the coffee machine. If you're honest with yourself, you'll know if she's intrigued by your wily charms.

Is She Not Interested?

Since the 1970s, Monica Moore, Ph.D., professor of psychology at Webster University in St. Louis, has spent countless hours studying the nonverbal signals women give off when they're interested in a man. And the ones when they're not.

Remember that you can't count on nonverbal communications to be a dictionary in which all behaviors mean the same thing for the same person. Think about the context, Dr. Moore says. But generally, she says, these are some of the more frequent warning signs that you should back off.

- She'll orient her body away from you.
- She'll nod less or not at all to your conversation.
- She'll stop looking you in the eye.
- She may cross her arms over her chest or cross her legs.
- She'll move her chair back from you.
- She'll stop smiling and may even frown.

Why can't she just say outright that she's uncomfortable? She's trying to spare your feelings, bud. "Women aren't little victims who can't say no," Dr. Moore says. "But it is very much the case that women in our culture have often been socialized to be more passive than men and to care for the feelings of others."

Making Your Move

Once you have established that the attraction is mutual, where do you begin?

Raise your sights. Remember that 1979 Bellamy Brothers hit, "If I Said You Had a Beautiful Body, Would You Hold It against Me?" Well, forget it. Those kind of pickup lines can get you slapped in a bar, and in trouble at work. "Keep the comments and compliments above the neck," says Rabin.

Question, but don't interrogate. Don't go barging into her personal life, asking things like her age, her marital status, her cup size. She'll let you know the things she wants you to know. By the way, asking appropriate questions is the hallmark of any good flirt, adds Rabin. It shows her that you find her truly interesting.

Don't lurk. Remember, no matter how interesting you may find her, you don't want to camp out next to her workstation or follow her from one exercise machine to the next at the gym. Flirting is a dance, says Rabin, but the dancers still need a rest from time to time. "If you don't push it and you don't go overboard, women will open up to you," she says.

Have fun. Flirting is more about enjoying a woman's company than a means to getting lucky, Rabin says. Sure, there's a subterranean sexual charge there. But it's not the focus of good flirting. "To let the joyful banter, the mystery, the wooing pass you by and go right for the kill is such a shame," she says. "It takes all the fun out of it."

Don't Cross the Line

It's no longer merely a matter of good manners for a guy to back off when a woman he's trying to flirt with sends out negative vibes. It's the law.

"Flirting is fun when both people want to participate," says Webster University's Dr. Monica Moore. "But when someone is flirting with someone who is giving very definite signals that this is not acceptable, then we're talking about sexual harassment."

Workplace sexual harassment claims are on the rise. In 1991, the U.S. Equal Employment Opportunities Commission (EEOC) reported 6,883 cases filed across the country. Just six years later, in 1997, that number more than doubled to 15,889. These days, what you say and do *can* be held against you in a court of law.

So when does innocent flirting cross the line into sexual harassment? According to the EEOC, if a woman's response to "unwelcome sexual advances, requests for sexual favors, and other verbal or physical conduct of a sexual nature . . . affects [her] employment, unreasonably interferes with [her] work performance, or creates an intimidating, hostile, or offensive work environment," *that's* sexual harassment.

As you can see, the law covers an awful lot of ground. It also doesn't require that the woman specifically notify you that what you're doing is unwelcome. You have to use your head here to keep your hinder parts out of hot water.

Drive a Woman Wild When You're Not in Bed

Romance has gotten a bum rap. If you think it's all about cloying novels with Fabio on the cover, boring English movies where nothing ever blows up, or fat little cherubs bouncing around, think again. It's really all about sex.

For starters, let's look at the root of the word. Romance is from the Latin *romanice,* meaning "in the Roman manner." All faults of ancient Rome aside, those boys had some major sex. And let's look at Cupid, the Roman god of erotic love. Today he's a pouty little pink bauble in dire need of a shot of testosterone. But he wasn't always such a wimp.

"Cupid was Venus's son," says Gregory J. P. Godek, author of the best-selling *1001 Ways to Be Romantic* and *Love: The Course They Forgot to Teach You in School.* "He had a bow he used to make people fall in love. And let me tell you, his bow was *big.*"

Nudge, nudge, wink, wink.

So if the mere mention of the word *romance* creates an overwhelming urge to power up your buzz saw, it's time to change your attitude. And not just for her sake.

"For crying out loud, it's about being selfish," says Godek. "You want to have more sex? Have more fun? Enjoy your days more? I'll tell you how to do it—be romantic." It's not just a matter of more sex, he adds. It's better sex. You see, how you treat a woman outside of the bedroom most definitely affects her inspiration in the bedroom.

The Passing of Passion

If you want a relationship full of what the French call *joie de vivre,* you need to know

about passion's Public Enemy Number One. "Routine can take the life right out of a relationship," says Carolyn Bushong, a licensed professional counselor in Denver and author of *Seven Dumbest Relationship Mistakes Smart People Make.*

Consider this: You wake up, shave, shower, and rush off to work. Nine or so hours later you return, scarf down a hurried dinner in front of the television, watch a few more shows, and head off to bed. You repeat this until you retire. Then, you have an extra eight hours to watch television.

And you want her to be thrilled by that? Not a chance. You're probably bored stiff, too, if you can wrest your eyes away from *Baywatch* long enough to admit it.

The cure? You guessed it—romance. Here's a crash course in the essence of tickling your sweetheart's fancy.

Be spontaneous. "Many women, when they say they want romance, mean spontaneity," says Godek. It's the unexpected that shocks and delights. The surprise trip, the fleeting kiss in the middle of yard work, the note on the bathroom mirror when she wakes up. Spontaneity, he adds, proves to her that you've been thinking of her when she least expects it.

Turn off the tube. Spend a week with the television off, suggests Godek. Not only will it spur you to action in other areas of your life, it'll free up time to spend passionately with your loved one.

Give the gift of unpredictability. If you bring her roses every Friday evening, that's not romance, that's clockwork. If you're stuck for an unpredictable gift idea, ask her girlfriends, sister, or mother, Bushong advises.

Take her car to work one day. Bring it back washed and with a box of chocolates on the seat, Godek suggests. Don't mention it to her. Let her find out when she goes to work the next day. Unless, of course, it's the middle of a sweltering summer. Then you might want to put the chocolates in the fridge.

Pretend you've just met. Plan a night at a club where you don't normally go, says Bushong. "Choose a wilder one, one very different from your normal habitat," she says. "Let her go ahead, wearing something a little slutty." You hang behind for a bit, letting the wolves hover around her, and then come to her rescue. This works anywhere, adds Bushong, even in places like the supermarket. You could accidentally bump into her in the produce section. As tempted as we are to make a melon remark, we won't. Bushong suggests the more subtle: "Could you tell me how to cook my cauliflower?"

Play Sherlock. One of women's biggest complaints, according to Bushong, is that men are stone-deaf when it comes to picking up clues. "When she says, 'Gosh, I love purple roses,' make a note. Literally, make a note." Surprise her with them later.

Be creative. We gave you a few pointers to get you started, but from here on it's up to you. "Everybody is amazingly creative. Everybody. You have wells of creativity in you," asserts Godek. Dip down into those wells and pull up a bucketful for her.

You see, when it's all boiled down, she only knows you love her by the things you do. "It ain't the feeling, it's the action," says Godek. "You have to take the action."

And, buddy, a little bit of action is worth a whole lot in the big picture. "Do you remember how good you felt at the beginning of your relationship?" asks Godek. "That's what it can still be like."

Let Her Miss You

Your goal is a passionate, exciting relationship. You would think that the more time you spend with her, the better.

Wrong.

Absence, said the seventeenth-century French writer Francois de La Rochefoucald, lessens the minor passions and increases the great ones, as the wind douses a candle and kindles a fire. Those aren't just the poetic words of a long-deceased duke—they apply very much today.

"You want to give her time to miss you," explains Carolyn Bushong, a licensed professional counselor. Absence breaks the routines that cripple so many couples' sense of romance. And it's just part of human nature to miss what you don't have.

But there's a caveat.

Gregory J. P. Godek, author of the best-selling *1001 Ways to Be Romantic*, tells the story of a young, self-made millionaire. In his mid-thirties, after largely ignoring his wife while he made his fortune, he decided to switch things around. He took off from work and decided to devote every waking moment to his wife.

"You know what he found out?" asks Godek. "You know what she wanted from him? About 27 minutes a day." Now that's 27 minutes of undivided attention, he notes, not just watching the news together. The point? She likes you around, just not all the time.

So take that separate vacation, plan that weekend apart, go out in the evening by yourself. Just make sure that when you are together, your attention is squarely where it belongs—on her.

Drive a Woman Wild with Words

Try this the next time you're having dinner with the parents of your partner: Stand up, clear your throat, and announce, "I am a wild, hairy love beast, and I want to ravage your daughter until she mews like a helpless kitten."

Didn't go over too well? Well, there are two reasons why. First, it's downright hokey. Second, it's about as appropriate as a Willie Nelson song in a French restaurant. But if you learn when sexy talk is appropriate and make good use of it, you will have in your possession a key to a magical realm.

"When a man voices the depths of his desire for a woman, it unleashes something in her," says Bonnie Gabriel, author of *The Fine Art of Erotic Talk: How to Entice, Excite, and Enchant Your Lover with Words*. Gabriel, who is based in San Francisco, also teaches a nation-wide seminar called The Magic of Making Love with Words.

Think your sweet pea just wouldn't be interested in something like dirty talk? Think again. According to *The Janus Report on Sexual Behavior*, men and women were virtually iden-tical in claiming dirty talk to be very normal or all right (58 percent of men and 57 percent of women). The problem is often just putting the right words in your mouth.

"A lot of men get performance anxiety on the verbal level," says Gabriel. "Because of that, they get tongue-tied. They make won-derful lovers on the physical level, but they don't use their voices."

Sure, about half of all women think dirty talk is just fine. But how do you know if the woman you're with is one of the other half? A few ill-chosen words in the heat of the night could quickly turn your close encounter into the big chill. Dirty talk is very much a double-edged sword, says Gabriel. The same words we use to express lust and excitement are often also used to degrade and abuse people.

Good news, says certified sex therapist Wendy Maltz. Women who like vociferous sex tend to also be vocal in requesting it. So, when you hear "talk sexy to me" or "I want to hear your voice" whispered in your ear, you need to be prepared. You need to spend some time now figuring out exactly *what* she wants to hear.

Aural Sex

In order to be a vocal virtuoso, it's im-portant to have a good handle on what sexy talk is all about. "For me, erotic talk is any kind of expression that arouses passion," says Gabriel. So now you know the goal: to arouse passion. Here's how to reach it.

Start slowly. You don't want to jump right in with the kind of words you find scratched above a urinal at a biker bar. "Most women have said that as much as they enjoy lusty talk, they would rather it wait until they are feeling very aroused before you get into the graphic stuff," says Gabriel.

Ask her what she likes. Use what Gabriel terms *erotic questioning*. During your lovemaking, try different things such as varying your caresses or changing the placement of your kisses. Then ask her which feels better.

Let her know how she's doing. Your partner wants to know if she's pleasing you. Speak up, suggests Gabriel. Not only is it sexu-ally stimulating to her but she'll also appreciate being appreciated. Tell her things like, "Yes, right there," or "Your touch is so incredible," or "I love it when you do that."

Create a safety zone. Tell your partner that you want to try an experiment. Spend some time just kissing and caressing, and then begin tossing out some phrases, words, and fantasies. Ask her if it increases the mood or dampens it. Make mental notes of the things she likes, and use them in the future. "This technique builds trust to the point where you can both really open up," explains Gabriel.

Keep an open mind. Say the two of you are happily ensconced in each others' voices. Out of the blue, she asks you to bray like a donkey. "Some people may have fantasies that turn the other person off," Gabriel says. The key here is to *never* mock or laugh at any of her fantasies. It will kill the trust you're working to develop. Instead, find a way to redirect her fantasy to something a little more palatable. Try saying something like, "Oh, what I'm really imagining is . . ." Or, if you manage it without wilting, go ahead and be Eeyore. "You can just take turns being there for each other if you can't find a common fantasy to build on," says Gabriel.

Take her flying. Many women love the imagery that comes with sexy talk, says Maltz. You can use your voice to take her on that magical trip. You might try telling her about the two of you together in the rolling waves, the scent of the tropics in the air. Describe the scene to her in intimate detail.

Reaping the Benefits

It's understandable if you're a bit shy about this erotic-talk thing. You're not alone. In the book *Just Married* by Barry Sinrod and Marlo Grey, the authors point out that 74 percent of women in the first two years of marriage say they're the chattier of the couple during sex.

But if you switch that around and become a master of bedroom banter, the rewards can be great. "Both partners benefit tremendously," says Gabriel. "It helps people open up a new side of their sexuality."

In other words, it's about turning your good girl bad. In the best way.

Reach Out and Touch Her

Sometimes fate, business trips, or an angry, stick-toting father can conspire to keep you away from the woman you love. That's when technology can be your friend.

"Phone sex is a wonderful way to keep the spark alive when you can't be together," says Bonnie Gabriel, author of *The Fine Art of Erotic Talk: How to Entice, Excite, and Enchant Your Lover with Words.*

Here, then, are some tips that Gabriel suggests you keep in mind when love is on the line.

Play off the fact that you're not there. Describe to her what you would do if you *were* there.

Book a trip to Fantasy Island. Dig around in the sexual closet for a while and pull out some of your favorite shared fantasies. Tell her how you imagine the two of you together in the fantasy.

Delve into the past. Talk throatily to her about things you've done together. Tell her how good it felt when she did that . . . or that . . . or especially *that.*

There's another avenue of long-distance communication that can work almost as well—computers. Chat rooms and instant messaging can provide you with a way to sweet-talk your lover without all the toll charges. Of course, says Gabriel, the sound of your voice is missing, so you'll have to adapt.

You'll need to be more descriptive to make up for the lack of sounds, Gabriel says. A good way to do that is to describe what your voice would otherwise convey. Tell her how you're moaning, how excited you are. With a little practice, you'll be as good as you are on the phone.

Practice is also the only way to get around that other difficulty of online sex—typing with one hand. "That can be a problem," admits Gabriel.

Compliment a Woman

Perhaps you consider yourself a pretty savvy investor. You have a few bucks tucked away in your retirement account. You keep a trained eye on the market and maybe even dabble a bit overseas.

Well, lend an ear, friend, because we're about to drop the hottest investment tip of your life on you. For a couple of seconds a day, we can make you rich beyond your wildest dreams. And you can't beat the price.

"If you give a woman the gift of a compliment, you're going to get back her love, respect, admiration, and devotion," reports Ellen Kreidman, Ph.D., a relationship expert and best-selling author of *Light His Fire* and *The 10-Second Kiss.* "Your cost? Nothing. Your reward? A woman who responds to your needs in return."

Sound like a pretty good deal? It is.

What Women Want to Hear

It's not necessarily your fault if giving compliments is a bit foreign to you. "Many men simply haven't learned what a woman wants to hear," Dr. Kreidman says. In relationships, we often unconsciously mimic what we saw in our own houses growing up. If your dad's idea of a compliment was grunting at the meat loaf your mom cooked, chances are pretty good you didn't take away a whole lot of valuable lessons from that. All is not lost, though—an old dog *can* learn new tricks. Here are a few things to keep in mind.

Say something. Anything. "When you say nothing, people always take it as a negative," says Dr. Kreidman. She got her hair cut? Pipe up. New dress? Sing out strong. "If you're

thinking that she already knows that you like the way she looks, the way she cooks, or that you're proud of her, it isn't enough. It has to be verbalized," she says.

Look for the little opportunities. There are countless ordinary occasions that are perfectly suited to a compliment, says Joan R. Shapiro, M.D., a Denver psychiatrist and coauthor of *Men: A Translation for Women.* "If you like the way she looks when she steps out of the car, say so," she says. Tell her what a wonderful mother she is. "That means a lot because we always doubt that."

Show her off to others. Complimenting her in front of other people is extremely powerful, no matter how much she shyly protests. "It's like when you got married and you said in front of everybody, 'I choose this woman,'" says Dr. Shapiro. "It's like saying it all over again."

"It always has three times the impact when you compliment her in front of other people," Dr. Kreidman agrees.

Keep the glow going. When she comes home from work beaming about something she has accomplished, it's because she wants to share it with you. "Express pride in her," Dr. Shapiro says. "Show her how impressed you are." Your opinion matters to her. Make sure she knows it.

Know her buttons. There are certain specifically female areas you need to be extra sensitive around. One is a woman's fear of getting older and less attractive to you. How many times has she asked you, "Honey, will you still love me when I'm old and wrinkled?" You probably joked around and told her, "No way, you're out the door for a 20-year-old." Bad move, says Dr. Kreidman. "She wants to hear how she grows more beautiful with every year that passes," she says.

Be her support team. If she's trying to overcome a personal problem like smoking or overeating, she needs you in her corner. Never, ever mock her attempts to better herself. "She really needs to hear how special she is for trying to improve herself," says Dr. Kreidman.

Make a game of it. Did she remember to put the cap back on the toothpaste? Did she remember to slide the seat back in your car so you don't have to cripple yourself getting in? Did she remember that you like crunchy, not smooth, peanut butter? Make a game of seeing how many small things you can notice about her, and point them out with a compliment.

Do it daily. "Don't let a day go by without taking time out to notice that wonderful woman," says Dr. Kreidman. "Compliment her every day on something she has done, who she is, or her physical appearance."

The Return on Your Investment

You have only two choices here—to criticize or compliment. Both start with the same letter but end far differently. Here's what happens when you criticize. "You'll have a woman who's unresponsive, cold, and unloving," says Dr. Kreidman. And you know what often happens then? "We fall in love because of the way we feel when we're with another person," she says. When a woman stops feeling beautiful and sexy and appreciated with a man, she's tempted to find those feelings elsewhere.

Here's what happens when you compliment. "A woman who feels good about herself when she's with you is automatically motivated to satisfy your needs and care about your feelings, and will try to please you," says Dr. Kreidman.

Tough choice, huh?

Instead of That, Try This

Her: "Do you love me?"

You: "Yup."

Bzzzzzz. You get zero points. Well, maybe a tiny fraction of one for at least answering in the affirmative. You see, questions like this one are your opportunity to shine, to really lay a sparkling compliment on her. It's all about being specific.

It's not enough to mutter generalities when you're complimenting the love of your life. You need hard-core detail. "It takes a little practice, but it's worth the extra effort," explains relationship expert Dr. Ellen Kreidman. "Sometimes a five-second compliment can make her feel wonderful for four hours." For example, instead of mumbling, "You look nice," try saying something like, "Wow, that red dress looks beautiful on you. It shows off your sexy legs," or "You're a knockout in that outfit. Every man at the party is going to envy me."

And what do you say after your wife or girlfriend has just cooked a delicious meal? Instead of muttering, "The dinner was good," tell your sweetie, "This is the best fried chicken I've ever tasted," or "That was terrific. I'm the luckiest man alive to be with such a fantastic cook."

Get the drift? Yes, it seems somewhat corny. That's because it is. But it shows her that she's so special to you that it moves you to hyperbole. She *wants* to be your apple tree blossom of a thousand perfumes.

And the answer when she asks if you love her? "I love you more than life itself. I can't imagine ever living without you. You mean everything to me," suggests Dr. Kreidman.

Unhook a Bra with One Hand

It was a moment of television brilliance.

In one of the early episodes of the series *Happy Days*, Fonzie was holed up in his 'office' at Arnold's. Next to him was his student for the day, Potsie. The lesson? How to unhook a woman's bra.

Potsie wrapped the bra around a radiator. The Fonz, with typical aplomb and a flexing of his leather-jacketed shoulders, sauntered over. Snap. With a deft turn of the wrist, and using only one hand, the bra fell to the floor.

Just a Hollywood trick shot? No way, says actor Henry Winkler, who portrayed the Fonz. It was a real bra with a real clasp. But Winkler is holding tight to the secret of his technique until his youngest son gets engaged. Until then, he lets slip with this helpful tidbit.

He asked bosom buddy Anson Williams (the actor who played Potsie) to hook the bra so that the clasp was directly over a ridge on the radiator. "I could use the ridge itself as a fulcrum," explains Winkler. From there you can note the similarity between a radiator ridge and a woman's spine—both provide the required leverage.

Success or Bust

If you're lucky, she's wearing a bra with a front clasp. "Those come off so easily. You can do it with one finger," says Cindy Cipriano, promotions director for Coquette Lingerie in Waterloo, Ontario.

If, on the other hand, you're faced with the ubiquitous back-clasper, Cipriano suggests a brief moment of Zenlike contemplation. "Relax. Don't rush it, and don't get frustrated," she says.

A typical bra uses a hook-and-eye clo-sure—and you need to envision how it works in order to unsnap it single-handedly, says Cipriano. Think of the bungee cord that you use to hold down the trunk of your car. It's elastic, it has a hook, and the rust hole that you wedge the hook into can be considered an eye. No matter how you tug, pull, or haul on it, it's going to stay put unless you back the hook out of the hole the same way it went in. The same is true of a bra.

According to Cipriano, here's what you need to do.

- If you're right-handed, nonchalantly let your right hand work its way around her to the clasp.
- Feel for the bump where the hook and eye meet.
- Place your thumb on one side of the bump, your forefinger and middle finger on the other.

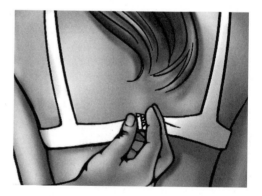

- Pressing against the strap, slide your thumb under your forefinger. It's kind of like snapping your fingers in slow motion.
- The clasp should slide apart. Remember, the straps are elasticized and may fly outward with some speed. Keep your face, eyes, and small items of furniture a safe distance away.

Don't sweat it if you miss the first time. It'll probably take a couple of tries. Once you get it, you'll wonder how there was ever a time when you didn't know how to do this.

Propose Marriage

Back in 1952, the heyday of male chauvinism, a Gallup poll showed that 82 percent of men popped the question when it came to proposing marriage, while only 9 percent of women did so. Forty-five years later, in 1997, Gallup asked the same question. The result? Identical.

It's doubtful anything else survived the women's liberation movement and the sexual revolution so perfectly intact, but there it is—proposing marriage is still a man's job.

You're up against some stiff competition. One man convinced the *New York Times* to imbed his proposal in one of its crosswords. Others have hired planes to pull banners behind with the big question. Billboard proposals are becoming increasingly popular. And one theatrical producer donned a cap and cape, bought 12 dozen roses, hired a 25-piece band, and rented a white steed to propose to his fair maiden with the royal entourage in tow.

Know When to Ask

There's a good reason for all these elaborate ways of asking what seems to be a simple yes-or-no question—it's not a simple yes-or-no question. In fact, it's probably the most important question of your life.

How you ask a woman to marry you is the first step in what, hopefully, is the grand adventure of your life. An exceptional proposal carries with it the promise of more magic to come. It gives her a delightful story to tell her friends, family, and children.

It reminds her, even in the darkest moments of a relationship, why she loves you so much.

One caveat: This is one question that you should only ask if you already know the answer. "If you're not 100 percent sure and it's something you haven't discussed before, I don't think there should be a proposal," says relationship expert Dr. Ellen Kreidman.

"Most men have a clear message from their girlfriends when they're ready," points out Dr. Kreidman. She'll talk about marriage, she'll talk about babies, she'll talk about the two of you in the future tense. If you're not sure, wait until you are. "You don't want to push someone into marriage," she says.

Popping the Question

Keep these hints from Dr. Kreidman in mind when you're pondering the big moment.

Be creative. "A really good proposal takes time and energy and effort," says Dr. Kreidman. "That's really the message that you're giving when you propose well." It's like buying a gift. If you run out Friday afternoon and buy her something off the rack at Chet's Bargain Basement, it shows. Same with a proposal.

Make it personal. We can give you examples like those above, but you're the one who really knows her. Build your proposal around something that she truly loves or enjoys. If she enjoys scuba diving, propose underwater with your waterproof pen and pad, surrounded by coral reefs. If she's a golfer, leave the ring and note in the cup at the 18th hole. You get the idea.

Stretch yourself. If you really want to impress her, do something that she knows is uncomfortable for you. If you hate the limelight, make your proposal very public. If you're normally as romantic as a stick, do something worthy of Valentino.

Don't stretch her. If she hates publicity, flashing your proposal on the jumbotron at halftime of the Super Bowl probably isn't a wise idea. "There are plenty of women who are shy and introverted and who would just die," says Dr. Kreidman.

Cook a Romantic Meal

If you labor under the misconception that the culinary arts are only for women and wimps, meet Biker Billy.

As comfortable on his Harley police bike as he is in the kitchen, Bill Hufnagle, host of the TV cooking show *Biker Billy Cooks with Fire* and author of a cookbook by the same name, scoffs at the idea that cooking is unmanly. "It's one of those myths," he says. "It's like the one that says all bikers are mean, evil people. It's not true."

So dust off your chopper and wipe the counter clean, it's time to learn the essence of creating a romantic meal for the apple of your eye. Because, as Hufnagle so eloquently puts it, "food is edible love."

Secrets of a Sensual Meal

The first secret of a romantic repast is simplicity. "A man needs to remember not to overdo it," says Martha Hopkins, coauthor of *InterCourses: An Aphrodisiac Cookbook.* "Anybody who thinks he's going to cook a five-course meal from scratch is out of his brain." Here's what you need to know if you want passionate sex on tonight's dessert menu.

Surprise her. Invite her over for, say, a movie. Or, if it's your wife, suggest a quiet game of cards in the evening. Then, when she walks in, she'll see that you've really been a cooking Casanova. "She'll love it," promises Hopkins. And you, too.

Plan ahead. Remember, the focus should be on your lady love, not the food. Cook what you can ahead of time, even the day before, says Hopkins. Don't try to do it all while she sits alone in the living room with a warming glass of wine, listening to your muffled curses.

Know what she likes. You may think your hot dog and peanut butter stew is the best dish since Betty Grable, but what if she doesn't like soup? Make a mental note of her favorites and also any allergies she has, Hufnagle suggests.

Choose a few choice dishes. Once you've established what she likes, select one or two dishes that you're going to make. Ideally, they are ones you've made before or ones that stand a reasonable chance of turning out on the first try. "You don't have to make a leg of lamb or some fancy French dish," Hufnagle says.

Augment your choices with premade dishes. "That's what the gourmet section in the grocery store is for," adds Hopkins. Get a dessert from a local bakery, appetizers from the Piggly Wiggly, and you're all set.

Set the mood. As important as the food you cook is the atmosphere you create. Candles or a crackling fireplace are always appropriate. "Fire captures the heat of the moment," says Hopkins. Appropriate music is another good bet. Even your clothes matter. If you're striving for a more formal meal, put a tie on under your apron.

Think presentation. Sorry, but a book *is* judged by its cover, and a Cornish hen by its glaze. Be artful in the way you serve the food, says Hufnagle. It doesn't matter how delightful your peppercorn sauce is if you serve it out of something from your army mess kit. If you make a salad, choose colorful vegetables. Nachos look wonderful with red bell peppers diced on top. Use parsley, kale, even wildflowers to garnish plates. Lay a breadstick on the side of the plate. Use your imagination, or steal some ideas from a magazine in the checkout line of the grocery store.

Go for aroma. Just like presentation, the way food smells is crucial to how she perceives it. When she walks in, the first thing that should greet her is a kiss from you. The second should be the smell of your cooking. Buy yourself some partially baked rolls at the grocery store, suggests Hufnagle. Throw them in the oven for a few minutes before she gets there. Consider choosing other foods that are as pleasing to the nose as they are tantalizing to the tongue. Baked Brie cheese, fresh spices, even crushed garlic scent the air wonderfully, he adds.

Be flexible. "A romantic meal can be so many things," says Hopkins. "Sometimes you feel really loving, sometimes you feel really playful, and sometimes you feel really horny. Pick the foods and moods to match." A picnic spread on the living room floor, an impromptu breakfast in bed, take-out food served with a candle and a glass of wine. They're all meals, they're all romantic.

"It's all about saying, 'I love you' with an act that includes food," Hufnagle says.

Wine and dine her. "Alcohol, if appropriate, is a good addition to almost any meal," says Hopkins. It relaxes the mood and adds to the ambiance. Choose the booze to suit the situation. Wine is almost always a good choice, as are after-dinner liqueurs. Don't overdo it, though. "If you have too much, the machinery isn't going to function," reminds Hopkins.

Forget about the dishes. Don't don your rubber gloves and leave her after a great meal. Forget about cleaning up and just concentrate on her, says Hopkins. The Joy you're looking for is not in a dish detergent bottle. There is a statute of limitations on this advice, however. Eventually, it's your job to clean up. Don't leave the mess for her to do later.

'A' for Effort

There are many ways to make your meal memorable, but remember one thing—the fact that you're doing it at all is significant. Don't sweat it if your cooking skills aren't completely up to par. "Women just love the fact that they're being cooked for," says Hufnagle. "It's really something they adore."

Eating for Pleasure

What makes a particular food sexy? Why are mangoes equated with lovers while corned beef hash just doesn't register on the lust-o-meter?

Martha Hopkins, coauthor of *InterCourses: An Aphrodisiac Cookbook*, has an interesting theory. Sensual foods, she says, should generally work as well on the body as they do on the plate. Here, then, are some of the foods she considers sexiest.

Honey. "The word rolls off your tongue," Hopkins says. "It's sticky, it's sweet. Picture the way it drips. You just keep drizzling it to wherever you want." But be cautioned—honey is not a lubricant, she stresses. It can gum up the works in a hurry if it's used that way.

Nutella. You know the stuff. It's a chocolate-hazelnut spread usually found in the peanut butter aisle. "We're all convinced it's just sex in a can," Hopkins says.

Grapes. Since the days of ancient Rome when Mark Antony fed grapes to Cleopatra, the juicy fruit has been associated with lovers. "The way they burst in your mouth is definitely sensual," she notes.

Oysters. What list of sexy foods would be complete without oysters?

Chocolate. "You can't mess up with chocolate," she says. But if you do, oh, what fun it is to clean up.

Asparagus. "A phallic symbol, albeit slender." Feed your lover steamed stalks of asparagus and watch her devour them.

Strawberries. Enough said.

So much so, adds Hopkins, that you may not make it to the end of the meal before she decides to put that strawberry sauce to another use. No problem. "Many meals taste better the next day," she says.

Give a Massage

Stand up. Look down for a moment. You will see an appendage of amazing erotic ability dangling at waist level. This member can take your lover to the heights of sexual ecstasy and to the inner depths of intimacy. It can arouse her yet also relax her. She loves it when it's in her hair or tickling the tip of her nose.

Of course, it's your hand.

Your hands have seen a lot. They've been the primary point of contact between you and the rest of the world. They've done your bidding at work, at home, at play. They've wiped the sweat from your brow, the blood from your skinned knee, the tears from your crying eyes. It's time to dust them off for yet one more assignment—the exquisite art of giving a massage.

Rest assured, you will be in the company of the finest of men. The father of Western medicine, Hippocrates, once wrote that "the physician must be acquainted with many things and assuredly with rubbing." The famous physician Galen also addressed massage techniques in his writings, 200 years after Christ. And one of the most common forms of massage—Swedish massage—was developed at the beginning of the nineteenth century by Swedish soldier and gymnast Per Ling. For his work, the king of Sweden bestowed honors upon Ling.

Two hundred years later, we're here to see to it that you're bestowed some honors in your own castle from your own queen.

Setting the Scene

The first thing you need to do is choose some appropriate oil, says Elliot Greene, a nationally certified massage therapist in Silver Spring, Maryland, and past president of the American Massage Therapy Association. Massage oils are readily available at health food stores, body boutiques, and even pharmacies, he says. Avoid mineral oil and baby oil, adds Greene; they are absorbed too quickly. "And, of course, avoid motor oil," he jokes. Just in case you were wondering.

Here are some additional tips for you to keep in mind.

Floor it. Chances are, you don't have a massage table. If you don't, Greene suggests stretching out a foam pad or a thick blanket on the floor. Make sure that it's something you don't mind getting a bit of oil on. Forget the bed. "It's too soft to support you properly," he says.

Trim your nails. Your partner's skin isn't the place to buff your fingernails. It's essential to make sure that they're cut short.

Notch up the thermostat. "When they're getting massages, people often become more sensitive to the room temperature," says Greene. Another option is to drape your partner in a sheet or towel and only expose the area you're working on at the moment. But what fun is that?

Notch down the noise. Turn off the television, disconnect the phone, and choose a time of day that's quieter. "You can have music that's soothing, if you like," says Greene.

Dim the lights. Turn off any overhead lighting and use soft incandescent bulbs. Candles also are a good choice.

Get some pillows. If you're kneeling on the floor and scooting around her body, chances are, your legs will begin to seize up on you, especially if they're generally tight. Greene suggests two thin pillows—one to kneel on, the other to put between your thighs and lower legs so that your heels don't drive into your buttocks.

Rubbing Her the Right Way

Now, let's get down to business. The first thing that you should bear in mind is that old Pointer Sisters song—"Slow Hand." There's a reason they sang it with such fervor. Women routinely complain that men are too hurried and too rough in their touching, notes Bernie Zilbergeld, Ph.D., a sex therapist in Oakland, California, in his book *The New Male Sexuality*. He writes that a gentle and slow touch is most often associated with intimacy and love. Remember that as you massage your mate.

We're going to give you a few tips to get you started, but bear this in mind—sensuous massage is a dance best choreographed through improvisation. Feel free to explore, caress, touch, alter. Ask her to speak up if something feels particularly good, if she wants you to concentrate more on a certain area, or if there's something she doesn't like, Greene says.

Following, then, are some basic massage techniques recommended by Greene.

Warm the oil in your hands. Nothing is crueler than having your lover nude before you in a peaceful, relaxed pose and then pouring cold oil on her skin. Cup your hand, fill it with a dab of oil about the size of a quarter (you don't want to put too much on— you can always add more) and warm it between your hands before you smooth it over the area you'll be working on.

Start gently. Before you start your massage, gently rest your hands on her. This acclimates her to your touch before you begin the actual work.

Stroke toward the heart. When you're working on her legs, that means your strokes will move upwards. On her arms, you'll stroke toward her body.

Learn to effleurage. The French gave us more than the Statue of Liberty—they also furnished us with

A Foot in the Rough

There are 52 bones in your feet, making up about a quarter of the number of bones in your body. Add to that 66 joints, 214 ligaments, 38 muscles, and a bunch of tendons, and you have a rough idea of how intricate your feet are. Topping that all off, women have about four times as many foot problems as men, likely a result of wearing high-heeled shoes so often.

No wonder it feels so good when you give her a foot massage.

Let's face it—nobody has the time to give a full-body massage as often as he (or she) would like. But, in a paltry couple of minutes, you can win your sweetheart's undying gratitude by massaging her aching feet.

Here's how, according to certified massage therapist Elliot Greene.

- Have your partner lie on her back on the floor. Provide some padding for comfort. Kneel or sit in front of her feet and apply some oil. Most feet don't need very much oil.
- Put your right hand flat on the sole of her foot, with the heel of your hand snug in the long arch. Use your left hand to hold her leg firmly just above the ankle. Slowly push your right hand into her foot, stretching her toes forward toward her knee. Hold for about 10 seconds.
- Then hold her heel with one hand and use the thumb of your other hand to make firm, small circles on the sole of her foot. Cover the entire sole with this motion.
- Work up to her toes by gently squeezing each one between your thumb and forefinger. Tug softly as you slide from the base of the toe right off the end.
- Finish by gently cupping her foot in both hands for a few moments, one hand on the bottom of her foot, the other on the top.

some words to describe massage strokes. Effleurage is the simplest of strokes and the one that should be used first to loosen her up. Basically, it's a light, long rhythmic stroke that adapts to each part of the body and generally runs with the grain of the muscle. On her legs, for example, use your cupped palms and gently glide upwards. In smaller areas like her neck, you can use the same stroke with just a finger or two. On her back, flatten your hands and broaden your strokes.

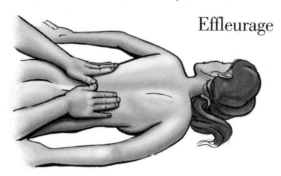

Effleurage

Play with petrissage. This is a stroke designed to squeeze the muscles and wring out toxins and tension. It works best on the shoulders, upper arms, legs, and buttocks. This stroke is circular, unlike effleurage. Use both your hands to work the muscles in opposite directions. When you're stroking her thighs, for example, your one palm or thumb will move away from you as you slide forward with it; the other palm or thumb will come toward you. You can use more pressure with this stroke to get down into the muscle, but always pay attention to the level of pressure with which your partner is comfortable.

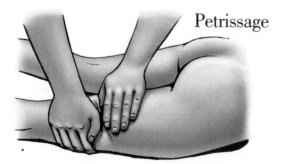

Petrissage

Roll your thumbs. Say she has a big old knot in a muscle. You'll be able to feel it as you become accustomed to touching her through massage. Thumb rolling is a good way to untie that knot. Use your thumbs one after the other, pressing into her flesh, sometimes moving circularly, other times just holding pressure on one point. If you lean your weight into this, you can turn it into a powerful massage movement.

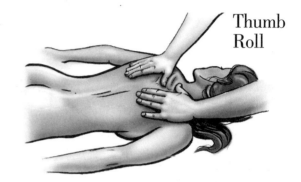

Thumb Roll

Give her face time. "People hold a lot of tension in their faces," says Greene. Use your fingertips in a gentle circular motion to massage the muscles in her jaw and around her temples. Also concentrate on her forehead from the eyebrows to the hairline. Be careful not to get oil in her eyes. A slight sheen on your hands will do.

Finish softly. Like a cooldown after a hard run, you want to end a massage on a gentle note. Feathering is a good way to do that. Use your fingertips to slowly stroke down your partner's back and gradually lighten the contact until your fingers are just stroking the air an inch above her skin.

Enjoy the afterglow. She's resting peacefully after your magical hands have worked their wonders. Let her enjoy it. Don't be in any rush to bring her back to the real world, says Greene. Drape her with a towel or blanket to keep her warm and just let her bask in the feeling. Don't worry, your thanks will come soon enough. When she does come down from the plane you've put her on, you'll see firsthand how appreciative she is. Now it's your turn to enjoy.

Part Seven

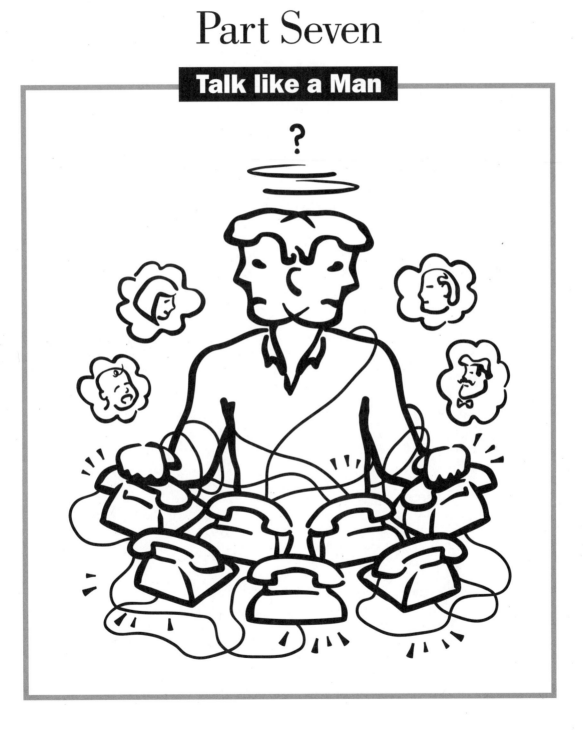

Get on the Air on Talk Radio

"Al from Altoona, you're on the air!"

If those are the words you pine to hear, well settle on in, tune your dial, and listen up. There are a few vital tricks to beating the others to the open line on a talk show. But the lessons don't stop there. Once you're on the air, what then? What makes the difference between a great caller and some boob who gets hung up on?

We'll tell you all that and more, but first, let's get you in the door ahead of all those other callers.

Let's Get Busy

It's no surprise that phoning a talk radio show rivals the federal government or an airline on Thanksgiving for busy signals. Demand for what talk radio is doling out is huge—in 1980, there were only 75 talk radio stations. By 1997, there were 1,250, with that number increasing by about 750 stations a year. And top talk radio hosts can have audiences the size of small countries. In the fall of 1997, Dr. Laura Schlessinger had 18 million listeners, with Howard Stern and Rush Limbaugh close behind with more than 17 million each.

So where does that put you? How can your anonymous little hand be seen waving over the sea of humanity? Take heart: Being in the unheard masses is actually to your advantage, says Travis Rodgers, producer of the *Jim Rome Show*, a nationwide sports-talk radio program.

Usually, Rodgers says, only about 2 percent of a show's listeners are trying to call in during any one show. "But the people we really want to hear from are the 98 percent who aren't calling." That's because the regular 2 percent of callers tend to be full of miscreants, the hopelessly unemployed, and the shiftless, he says. They're the ones with the extra time on their hands.

But there are ways to get on the air without spending a huge chunk of your workday getting busy signals. Rodgers offers these tips.

Call early. Jim Rome's show, for example, starts at 9:00 A.M. Pacific time. They start taking calls at 9:15. Call 5 or 10 minutes before the show you listen to starts picking up. Just let it ring. Nobody is going to hang up on you. If you're at work, put it on speakerphone and go about your business until you hear someone answer.

Learn how to dial. "Our phone lines are always busy. We never have an open line for more than 5 to 10 seconds," explains Rodgers. But those few seconds are actually a window into the show if you use them correctly. Remember this—most shows are on a 7-second delay. That gives the producers a chance to beep out anything too crass before it goes out on the air. So when you hear a caller on the radio start to wrap up his comments, odds are that he has actually just finished. Dial like crazy when you hear him summing up, and you can often grab that newly opened line.

Have something interesting to say. "If you do, you're going to get put right at the top of the line," says Rodgers. "I want to hear it as much as I want my audience to hear it." Most times you call a talk radio show, you'll get someone like Rodgers screening you. They want to know what you're going to say. "Very few people have thought it out carefully," he says. "They have a germ of an idea, but then they get on and stammer and sound like an idiot." Make sure that you turn that germ into a full-fledged plague before you call, or the next sound you hear will be a dial tone.

You're on the Air

Congratulations. You made it through, and now you're going to be able to speak your piece to thousands or even millions of listeners. Obviously, you don't want to sound like a bozo. To help you out, we went to Ray Suarez, host of National Public Radio's news talk show *Talk of the Nation*, which is broadcast to more than 120 stations nationwide. Here's how to sound good in front of your countrymen.

Realize that you're welcome. Some talk radio shows can get a little vicious, but without the callers, they're nothing. "When the callers are terrific, the show is terrific," says Suarez. "I can be Mr. Bon Mot, Mr. Amazing, Oscar Wilde Junior, but if the callers suck, the show sucks. Callers drive the show."

Get to the point. Sometimes, out of nervousness or servility, callers will spend the first few minutes waxing poetic over how much they love the show, love the host, love the lint on the host's britches. "They're wasting my time," says Suarez. "I realize they feel it very sincerely, but the clock is a tyrant."

On talk radio, brevity is the soul of wit. So don't be a half-wit. Be brief.

Ask and ye shall receive. Callers don't need to offer some outstanding insight that nobody in the world has ever thought of before— they just need a valid question. If you're reasonably intelligent and the show has made a question linger in your mind, go ahead and ask it. "Good questions help thousands of other listeners who were wondering the same thing," notes Suarez.

Go with what you know. What happens if the topic of the day is something that you don't know squat about? Tie it into an area you are knowledgeable in, says Suarez. Say the topic is why the United States had to maintain a military presence in Bosnia for so long. Only problem is, you couldn't find Bosnia on a map if your life depended on it. "But Haiti is your meat and potatoes," says Suarez. "You could ask, 'What's the difference?' We saw terrible things in Haiti but still got out right away."

Know when to stop. You don't want to end a good call by blathering on until someone hangs up on you. Say what you have to say,

Strange New World

With talk radio undergoing a meteoric rise in popularity, it's only natural that a few new idiosyncrasies should emerge. But whole new languages? Well, pretty close. Several shows have certainly adapted the English language in novel ways.

On the *Jim Rome Show*, a Los Angeles–based sports-talk radio program heard across the country, a whole glossary of terms is necessary to keep you in the know when listening. What do you expect from a show with the motto "Have a take. Don't suck!"? A take, of course, is something worthwhile to say.

When in Rome, here are some other lingual aberrations to keep in mind.

To bag someone out: To criticize

Barry Manilow: Joe Montana, for his physical resemblance

Brick: A New Yorker, or a New York Knick; also anything East Coast in origin, for the number of brick buildings in the area as well as for the Knicks' tendency to shoot bricks

The incident: Jim Rome's physical confrontation with former Rams quarterback Jim Everett after repeatedly calling him Chris Evert, in reference to the female tennis player; comes from Rome's reluctance to discuss—you guessed it—"the incident"

thank the host, and stop. "Or else the host will make you stop, and that's just not as nice," says Suarez. Many callers tend to go through their spiel and, once finished, start right back at the top of the loop again. It's not more convincing the second time around.

So, thank you, dear reader. It was a pleasure. Hope to do it again soon.

See how it's done?

Survive an IRS Audit

Vasectomies performed by a lumberjack. Shaving with a dull toenail. Grunting out a very large peach pit. All have about the same fun factor as an IRS audit.

So know this: The way you talk to and treat an agent of the Internal Revenue Service can make the process at least bearable, if not exactly pleasant. If you approach the IRS agent as a human being instead of as the henchman of a corrupt and evil empire, you may just find a cooperative, reasonable person underneath the stigma associated with the job.

Agents of the IRS are usually consummate professionals, says Charles H. Mansour, a Houston tax lawyer at Mansour and Associates. When taxpayers run into difficulties, it's often because of a personality conflict.

Here's how to help things go smoothly.

Taxing Your Patience

The first thing you need to determine is if the audit is legal. In most cases, you must be informed of an audit within three years of the time you filed your return. Once in a while, the IRS fouls up and sends you a notice after the statute of limitations has expired. You can have this audit thrown out in court. If this happens, consult a tax professional. If it is legit, Mansour suggests you keep these tips in mind.

Reschedule, if necessary. If you know you won't be ready in time, contact the agent listed on the audit notice and request a postponement. "They will generally oblige," says Mansour.

Be organized. A sure way to tick the agent off is to bring your receipts and canceled checks to him in a lunch box. File them according to category. For example, have both receipts and checks for office supplies in one file.

Be courteous. It's understandable if you resent having to justify yourself to the IRS. Just don't let the agent know that you do. "They have immense power. You want to minimize the chance of any personal animus getting into the process," says Mansour.

Put out the welcome mat. Show the agent where the coffeepot is. Point out the rest room. Give him a quiet place to work out of the fray of work or home. But make sure that's all you offer. Don't try to foist some scotch or a first-born daughter on him in the hopes that he'll go easy. And don't even think about trying to ply him with C-notes. "It is absolutely, completely illegal. You would be very foolish to do that," says Mansour.

Record the interview. If you give the IRS advance notice, you can record any conversations you have with the agent. This ensures that they play by the book. "Most agents do not inject personal issues into an audit, but this eliminates the possibility," Mansour adds.

Speak only when spoken to. You thought you outgrew that, right? Not in this case. Just answer the questions the agent asks.

Don't guess or surmise. If the agent asks something you're not sure of or don't know, tell him you'll get back to him with an answer. When he leaves, he'll give you an itemized list of information he needs or questions he needs answers for. By not answering, you avoid giving him wrong information that can cause you grief down the road.

The IRS is making great strides in becoming more taxpayer friendly, says Mansour, but that still doesn't mean you have to put up with shoddy treatment. If your courtesy ultimately fails and the agent treats you unfairly, don't take any bull. "My advice is to always be nice, but if you do not feel that you're being treated adequately, ask to speak to his manager," says Mansour.

Even evil henchmen have bosses.

Talk Your Way out of a Traffic Ticket

James Bond with a speeding ticket? Not a chance.

In 1996, actor Pierce Brosnan spent some time filming a movie in Wallace, Idaho, where he developed a well-deserved reputation for having a lead foot. Four times, the local constabulary pulled him over for speeding in the same BMW Z3 convertible he used in the 007 flick *Goldeneye*. And four times, they let him off without a ticket.

Sure, fame helps. So does having a newly released sweetheart of a car that the cops will drool over. But talking your way out of a ticket isn't all German engineering and superspy charm—there are techniques that we Joe Blows can use to increase our chances of leaving a roadside stop with just a warning.

Getting Out of a Fine Mess

Here are some tried-and-true tactics, courtesy of Mark D. Sutherland, a traffic ticket attorney in Santa Ana and Northern California and coauthor of *Traffic Ticket Defense*.

Pull over as far as you safely can. For you to have any chance of driving away ticketless, you need the police officer to feel comfortable enough to spend a few minutes talking to you. If he's worried about becoming road pizza, he's not going to hang around at your window.

Make him comfortable. Likewise, you have to convince him that you're not a dangerous criminal. "Every cop worries at every stop that he's going to get shot in the face," says Sutherland.

Remain seated, roll your window down,

and place both hands on the steering wheel. If it's night, turn on your interior light. Never reach down to the right for anything. All he sees from behind the car is you reaching for something that could be a gun.

Be cooperative. "You may not be able to talk your way out of a ticket all the time, but you sure as hell can talk your way into one," says Sutherland. Don't even think about trying to intimidate the cop by saying something like, "Oh yeah? I'll see you in court." He may just hunt for another infraction to pop you with. "If I see more than one charge on a ticket, I can always tell the driver copped an attitude," Sutherland says.

Can the excuses. They generally don't work. If you whine that this ticket will cause you to lose your license, you're guaranteed to get one.

Additionally, the following excuses spell certain doom: "But, officer, my speedometer is acting up." "I really had to take a leak and was hunting for a bathroom." "Sorry, I'm late for work." Forget them. About the only legitimate excuse is a medical emergency.

Don't incriminate yourself. Often, the cop will ask you, "Do you have any idea how fast you were going?" If you say yes, it's an admission of guilt. If you say no, you look dumb. Try this line, suggests Sutherland: "Okay, officer, if I get this right, will you not write me a ticket?" Who knows? He may agree. If he doesn't, at least you've given him a chuckle and maybe he'll let you off anyway.

These tips will help your chances of not getting a ticket. But if the cop has a quota to make or is just in a surly mood, you'll likely get one. In that case, look around for things that will help you get it tossed out in court. Are any speed limit signs missing? Where was he when he nailed you?

Jot anything even slightly relevant down and take it to court. If you're prepared, you can often get the ticket thrown out or the fine reduced, Sutherland says.

Be Your Own Lawyer

Sleazy lawyer jokes aside, who wouldn't prefer to hand the burden of a court case to a trained professional? Unfortunately, with lawyer fees ranging in the area of $150 per hour and up, sometimes you just can't afford it.

That's what a small claims court is for. As its name suggests, it's a forum for settling monetary disputes under a certain amount. It is, says Edward I. Koch, former mayor of New York City and judge on the television show *The People's Court*, a lawyer-free zone. You must represent yourself there.

While small claims court is the most obvious exception, there are times when a man who represents himself truly does have a fool for a client. Like in a criminal matter. "You always ought to have a lawyer if you are involved in any capacity in the criminal courts," says Koch, who is also a partner in the New York City law firm Robinson, Silverman, Pearce, Aronsohn, and Berman.

Likewise, if a case doesn't involve money, you're often better off getting a real legal eagle, says Paul Bergman, professor of law at the University of California, Los Angeles, and coauthor of the book *Represent Yourself in Court*. Cases that involve property rights, custody disputes, and the like can get pretty tricky, he explains—often beyond the skills of most do-it-yourselfers.

Going to Court

Small claims is a concept as well as a court name. In some states, the venue is simply called small claims court. In others, it goes by a different name but has a similar function. Your small claims case may be heard in municipal court or district court or county court. To top it off, each state has different maximum amounts you can sue for in a small claims case, ranging from $2,000 in New Jersey, $3,000 in New York, and $5,000 in California, to $10,000 in Maryland. Call the mayor's office in your city to find out how to contact your local small claims court, Koch suggests.

Once you have paid your filing fees and lodged your complaint, it's time to do some homework. Here are a few things for you to keep in mind.

Be Joe Friday, not Perry Mason. For small claims court, it's not necessary to hit the law libraries seeking out historic judgments, legal precedents, and obscure statutes. "The judge knows the law. Let him worry about that," says Koch. "It's the facts that count."

Befriend the court clerk. "They try not to give legal advice, but they can be very helpful," Bergman says of court clerks. From giving you help with filing forms to filling you in on court policies, the clerk can be a valuable ally.

Write it out. When you sit and commit your case to paper, you're doing yourself a big favor. "In writing it out, you become more familiar with all the facts, and you can decide what you want to highlight," explains Koch.

You would do well to even come up with a trial notebook, suggests Bergman. In it, you outline what you need to prove and what evidence you need as well as lists of names, numbers, dates, and other pertinent facts. Consider it your courtroom manager.

Get the documents. Any written receipts, any disputed bills, any lease forms—dig them out. "The first question most small claims court judges will ask is 'Do you have any documentary evidence?'" says Bergman. If you've been involved in a fender bender and are seeking damages, you better have a repair estimate. Don't even think about giving the judge your opinion on what you figure it will cost. "Forget it, judges aren't going to want to hear that," cautions Bergman.

Sit in on other cases. Pack yourself a lunch and plan to spend a few hours at the courthouse listening to other cases. Ideally, you'll want to sit in on the judge who will be hearing your case. Get a feel for the way things work, the questions the judge asks. Try to hear at least five different cases, Bergman suggests.

Be organized. Don't bring your case to court in a shoe box, advises Bergman. Have everything filed and easily accessible.

Dress for the part. "Don't come to court schlumpy," says Bergman. Small claims court is intended to be a little more casual, but it still is a court of law. Reflect that in your dress. "You don't have to dress as though you're an aristocrat, but you want to show respect for the system," says Bergman. A sport coat and tie are always suitable. Relaxed business attire is okay, too. Just make sure everything's pressed and clean.

Misrepresenting Yourself

Unfortunately, the facts do *not* always speak for themselves. You have to represent them. This can be a problem if you do and say things that can sabotage your case. Here are some of the worst mistakes you can make when representing yourself.

Running at the mouth. "They talk too much," Koch says of a commonly made error. "They're all over the map instead of concentrating on what the real issue is so that, occasionally, their best points are lost."

Being polite to the "little lady." If you have a woman judge, never refer to her as "ma'am," says Bergman. It's always "your honor" or "judge."

Dissing the judge. In a court, you never speak directly to your opponents. Always direct your comments or questions to the judge, suggests Bergman.

Do You Have a Case?

Before you take any legal gripe to small claims court, it's a good idea to determine if you stand a fair chance of winning. What's the point of spending the time and money if your complaint is gratuitous or doesn't have a legal leg to stand on?

So how do you know? "Generally, only a lawyer can tell you that," says Edward I. Koch, who is the judge on the television show *The People's Court*. If you're not sure your case has merit, spend the money on a consultation with a lawyer and have him look it over. It can also save you some embarrassment.

Take the case of Paul Shimkonis. In 1998, the Florida man sued a topless dancer and a strip bar. After originally being filed in Pinellas County circuit court, the suit eventually made its way to Koch's televised small claims court. Shimkonis's complaint? He said he was injured when Tawny Peaks slammed her 69HH breasts into his head.

While most of us would gladly be pummeled into a semiconscious stupor in such a fashion, Shimkonis asked Koch to award him suitable damages. Koch declined, ruling that he wasn't convinced any injury had occurred.

So, you see, it pays to keep abreast of the law.

Dissing the clerk. "One of the biggest things you can do to tick off the judge is to somehow get the clerk mad at you," says Bergman. "If it's a matter of who the judge is going to pacify—you or the clerk—it's going to be the clerk." Remember when we told you to befriend the clerk?

Saying the wrong thing. Want to impale yourself on the sword of justice? Tell the judge, "Don't interrupt me." That, says Koch, will do it every time.

Handle Telephone Solicitors

Some things are universal. The need for oxygen. The confusion over why women like Kenny G. The temptation to actually buy one of those checkout tabloids that creeps up before your principles kick in. The loathing directed toward telemarketers.

Yes, they do always call while you're eating your evening pork and beans. That's because they know that you're likely to be home then. But, as satisfying as it may be to disparage the lineage and offspring of telephone solicitors, you're not helping your aim of receiving fewer calls. To keep them from interrupting future reruns of *Star Trek*, you're better off following the advice of Beth Givens, director of the Privacy Rights Clearinghouse in San Diego, a nonprofit organization devoted to privacy issues, and author of *The Privacy Rights Handbook: How to Take Control of Your Personal Information*.

Turn Down the Volume

There are a number of ways telemarketers get your number. Some go through the phone book. Others have random dialers that cover all possible numbers. When you sign up for a contest, it's often a ploy to collect names and numbers. Printing your phone number on your checks is another good way to let the telemarketing world know you're there. Avoiding these practices can help you in the future.

But that doesn't help when the phone is ringing and your temper is rising. Employ these tactics from Givens.

Launch a preemptive strike. Send a letter requesting removal of your name from all lists to Telephone Preference Services, Direct Marketing Association, P.O. Box 9014, Farming-dale, NY 11735-9014. This will reduce calls substantially.

Don't hang up. When Cyndi starts nattering away about why you should switch your phone service, it's tempting to just slam down the phone. Don't. When you do that, she'll just note that you were at home at that time, and she'll call you back in the days to come.

Put yourself on the list. Immediately say, "Please put me on your don't-call list." Federal law requires them to maintain such a list and forbids them from calling again. Write down the rep's name, the company, its phone number, and the date of the call. If the company calls again, you can sue for up to $500 per call. Bear in mind that nonprofit fund-raisers and research surveys are exempt from this rule, but the better ones still maintain these lists.

Never buy anything over the phone. If you do, your name may go on a "sucker list." The fact that you bought puts you at the top of the list, and the company will also sell that information to other companies. Plus, scam artists love to buy those lists because it shows that you may be more easily duped. If you're genuinely interested in what the telemarketer is selling, ask him to mail you written materials explaining the offer. If he refuses, the company is probably not reputable.

Get off the phone. You've probably heard and read lots of stories about how people told telemarketers off in lengthy, elaborate ways. Don't bother. The longer you spend on the phone with them, the greater the chance of being sold something. Just say your piece and go back to sopping up your gravy.

Never divulge personal information. If you do get sucked into listening or taking part in a survey, never give out highly specific information. If the telemarketer wants to know your birth date (year of birth is okay), social security number, credit card number, or bank account number, hang up pronto. Scam artists can use this information to do things like apply for credit in your name or make withdrawals from your bank accounts.

Handle Pushy Salesmen

Even if you're buying new, it's understandable if you feel a little used.

You are far from alone. Since 1977, the Gallup Organization has been asking Americans to rate 26 different occupations for their "honesty and ethical standards."

For an unblemished 20 years in a row, from 1977 to 1997, one group had the dubious honor of finishing dead last in the survey. No, not lawyers. Not even politicians.

Car salesmen. The Pinto-pushers were rated so low that, in 1997, they were the only occupation to have a majority of Americans call their ethical standards "low" or "very low." Insurance salesmen didn't do a lot better. They were second-to-last over the 20-year period, with congressmen just above them.

Whether it's term life or tubeless tires you're haggling over, the methods of dealing with pushy salesmen are the same. Remember, you don't have to put up with obnoxious behavior from someone who's trying to get his hands on your money. It's important to note that the guy in front of you is being more aggressive than Roseanne around a pork chop because he thinks it's effective.

"Maybe his mannerism has worked for him a hundred times, but this is you, and this is a potential sale," explains Jeff Davidson, a certified management consultant in Chapel Hill, North Carolina, and author of the *Complete Idiot's Guide to Assertiveness*.

The Confident Consumer

Here are some tips that Davidson offers to keep you from getting steamrollered into a purchase you don't want to make.

Be honest. Tell him right away that you're uncomfortable with his pace and that you won't make a purchase if you're pressured. "You help break him out of his sales mode and get him back to being a person again," says Davidson.

Decommission him. Car salesmen, appliance dealers, computer reps, real estate agents, and many others work on commission. They're the ones who tend to be pushiest because if you go home empty-handed, so do they. Make it clear that the sale depends on the way they treat you. You'll be amazed at how quickly they undergo a personality change.

Beware the time-limited offer. Davidson had a roofing salesman in his living room attempting to give him the fast sell. The contractor was armed with various quotes, figures, and timelines. But the roofer wanted an answer right away so he could "schedule his people." Hey, you're the one with the money. It's not up to you to work around his schedule. "I told him that if he needed an answer right away, then it was no," says Davidson. Amazing how that schedule freed up.

Get somebody else. If he just won't back off, politely ask for another sales rep. If you want, you can do it under the guise of wanting to speak to someone closer to you in age or interests or whatever.

Tell him off. If all else fails, tell the guy to take a hike, says Davidson. "You don't have to stand for the tactics you're being subjected to," he says. Playing the heavy is not fun, but neither is being pushed around.

Cool off. If you do get sucked in, federal law gives you three days to back out of the sales agreement in certain circumstances. It's called the cooling-off rule. If the pitch was made by a door-to-door salesman at your home or work or a rented location, such as a hotel or convention center, the seller must give you notice that you have until midnight three business days later to cancel orders or purchases of $25.00 or more. Some exceptions apply, notably to tent sales by car dealers who have permanent locations somewhere else. For full information, contact the Federal Trade Commission.

Put It in Writing and Get Results

When you get stuck with a tainted gimcrack or a faulty whoosit, you could call up the customer service department and bark at the minimum wage–earning phone operator. But it's not your best option. First of all, some companies require that you state your case in writing right from the outset. Secondly, putting it in writing provides a paper trail if you end up having to settle the issue in court.

Here are some tips to keep in mind from Holly Cherico, vice president of communications for the Council of Better Business Bureaus, which is the headquarters of nationwide Better Business Bureaus, located in Arlington, Virginia.

Do it now. "The sooner you can get started, the better," says Cherico. If you wait, memories fade and warranties expire.

Get it together. Gather all relevant documents to your complaint, like receipts, repair estimates, whatever. Make copies and include them with your letter. Never send originals.

Be cool. "It never behooves anybody to be belligerent," explains Cherico. It's understandable that you're a bit hot under the collar, but you can sink your own ship by being an ogre. "The company is going to think they've lost your business anyway if you're nasty," adds Cherico.

Be positive. Conversely, if you put in a line or two about how you have been a longtime customer and have recommended them countless times, the company is more likely to bend over backward for you.

Go to the top. Address your letter to the president of the company. You can get his name by checking out the company's Web site, if it has one. Or just call and ask. If it's a large company, it's doubtful he'll actually see it. Bill Gates doesn't sift through mail from people whining about his latest overpriced software release. But his office staff will pass it to the people who will look after it. And it's coming from the top instead of the bottom. "When you get something from the president, you take extra care," points out Cherico.

Keep it simple. Make your requests in straightforward, easy-to-understand terms. If they have to wonder what planet you're from, it takes away from the message you're trying to get across.

Mail it certified. This gives you the paper trail mentioned earlier. You'll have a record of who received your letter and when.

Set a deadline. Be sensible here. Don't insist on a Wednesday response when it's Tuesday evening. "Ten business days is certainly reasonable," says Cherico.

When you send your letter, file a copy with the Better Business Bureau in your area. If the complaint doesn't pan out, they can investigate it for you and try to seek a solution.

"Most of the time, we can resolve it with a phone call," says Cherico. Plus, if you're dealing with a sleazy outfit, the Better Business Bureau can warn other consumers. Consider it your civic duty. And the good thing is that it's cheaper than cheap. "The Better Business Bureau handles this at no charge," says Cherico. That's definitely a better deal than you got on the product you're trying to return.

If it's a case dealing with what appears to be fraud, you should also contact your state's attorney general or local consumer protection office.

Remember, you already got sucked in once. Don't double the pain by running to one of those professional complaint-handlers who charge a fee for what the Better Business Bureau and others do for nothing. "I see no need for that until you've tried the nonprofit route first," says Cherico.

Raising Your Standard

When you're writing a letter of complaint, it helps to follow a standardized format. That way, you make sure you've covered everything. The following complaint letter is structured according to the Better Business Bureau's recommendations. The content, however, is distinctly ours.

Date
January 1, 2000

(Your Address)
Harry Harried
123 Misery Lane
Sorrowtown, U.S.A.

(Their Address)
Fred Fatherinlaw
Stork Industries
1000 Baby Lane
Maternity, U.S.A.

Re: Your product

Dear Mr. Fatherinlaw:

(State the Facts)
On or about (I always forget) June 30, 1982, I purchased your Michelle Anne model, serial number 091261, in an elaborate ceremony at St. Luke's. This model has several options, including a dual electronic reverb unit with a sonic capacity of 230 decibels. As your records likely show, it was the buy-now-pay-later plan.

(State the Problem)
I have no complaints with either the structural integrity or cosmetics of the unit. In fact, it buffs up nicely. However, I wish you had given greater care to the internal wiring of the unit. It does not respond well to spoken commands and will often even do the exact opposite of what you tell it. In addition, certain voice commands cause the unit to emit fiery sparks and exceed the 230-decibel limit.

(State What You Want the Company to Do)
To resolve the problem, I am asking for an extended maintenance plan whereby I would return the unit to your factory for several weeks a year for a tune-up. I must warn you that, when packed for shipping, the unit now includes two smaller subsidiary units with their own sets of idiosyncrasies.

(Apprise the Company of Your Time Frame and How to Contact You)
I look forward to your reply and fervently hope that I receive your permission to send the units packing next week. In the meantime, I can be contacted at the above address or in the back booth of Ned's Neighborhood Bar.

Sincerely,

Harry Harried

Make Small Talk

If you find making small talk painful, just be glad you're not a dog. Dogs sniff each other's butts to accomplish the same basic social function.

"A dog is simply trying to identify the other dog," says Mark L. Knapp, Ph.D., professor of speech communication at the University of Texas in Austin and author of *Interpersonal Communication and Human Relationships.* "We're doing that in small talk, but we're also doing much more."

Small talk, though it has a diminutive name, actually serves a big purpose, says Dr. Knapp. "It's a proving ground for a new relationship," he explains, whether it be romantic, social, or business-related. Fortunately, he adds, at the beginning of a new relationship, we generally give each other the benefit of the doubt. It's up to you to let the other person know, through what you say, if you're a putz or a pretty good guy.

If we turn out okay, we move on to the next stage of the relationship, whether it's going out for a beer, closing a deal, or asking for a date. "Both parties are saying, 'Here's a chance we might have. Let's explore more,'" says Dr. Knapp.

Your ability to make small talk can also mean the difference between getting a job and not, according to Barbara A. Kent, assistant director of the management communications program at Stanford University's Graduate School of Business. More and more job interviews are done partially over lunch or in some other social setting, she explains. "That's so the boss can see how you would interact with clients and others in the company. That's your chance to really impress him."

Making Small Talk Big

There's a lot riding on the ability to make small talk, but for some reason many guys hate doing it. "They see it as trivial or unimportant," says Dr. Knapp. It also may be as simple as the fact that they're just not very good at it.

So we culled advice from some of the people who know the most about making small talk. Here's what they said.

Throw the change-up. On every show, Alex Trebek, host of the TV game show *Jeopardy!*, spends a few minutes making small talk with the contestants. The secret to good small talk, he says, is to get people out of their rigid mindsets.

"Just pick something that throws them off a little, but that they're still able to talk about," he recommends. "Something like, 'I understand you're an ax murderer, but you got off. Tell me what happened.'" Then, when they've told you the story, pick up another thread of it and continue. "Do you plan to throw axes again in competition?" suggests Trebek.

Pass the bar. Bartenders spend a lot of time making small talk. It's a big part of the job description—not to mention their tips. So how do bartenders strike up a conversation? They get you to talk about your favorite subject: you. "People love talking about themselves," says Karl Kozel, a bartender at Manhattan's ultrachic Gotham Bar and Grill. "You just need to coax it out a little."

A great way to start is to inquire about a guy's hometown. It's generally a place he feels passionate about. From there, you can look for connections. Have either of you been in the same places? Have you met any of the same people? And if you find yourself wearying, do what Kozel does. Introduce him to somebody else nearby. Then there's another person who can toss in his two cents. "That takes a little of the pressure off you," says Kozel.

Take a date. Women and men approach small talk very differently, says Kent. Men use it to get on to the next, more comfortable stage of knowing someone. Women get more pleasure just from the casual banter. They're not in as much of a rush to leap to the next stage. If you tire of the pleasantries, stand back and let your lady take over.

See eye to eye. Larry Fila Jr. is director

of the Maryland Barber School and a longtime barber himself in Brooklyn Park, Maryland. He's made a lot of small talk. And, he says, it's essential to keeping customers coming back. Good small talk, he explains, begins from the first moment you lay eyes on someone. So you need to get on the same eye level. If you're both standing, no problem. If he's sitting, sit next to him. "It's intimidating when you're looking down on him," says Fila. Flashing your best Mr. Nice Guy smile also helps put the other person at ease.

Make contact. When you first meet another guy, Fila suggests a handshake or a clap on the shoulder. From there, he says, you should listen twice as much as you talk. "If you give him the opportunity to open up, it'll really start clicking," says Fila. At the end of the conversation, thank him. Say how much you enjoyed talking. "Let him know that he's appreciated." It will make it much easier the next time you see him.

Small Pleasures

When all is said (or not said) and done, you have a choice. You can turn a cold shoulder to the art of small talk and be miserable. "It's not a lot of fun for two people to stand there in un-comfortable silence," says Dr. Knapp.

Or you can embrace it.

Men like it when they're com-fortable in relationships. They like being able to wisecrack with their pals, have coffee with their clients, be cozy with their wives. But you're never going to get to that stage until you go through the gateway of small talk first. And you're always going to be in the situa-tion of standing next to somebody new.

Why not enjoy the process?

How to Kill 10 Minutes with Someone You Hate

Next time you find yourself next to the one person you loathe most, try these tips courtesy of Amy Mills Tunnicliffe, director of the Proper Manner, a corporate etiquette and business skills consulting company in Hingham, Massachusetts.

Make the first move. "Suck it up, take a deep breath, and put a smile on your face," Tunnicliffe says. That way, you don't have to spend the rest of your time dreading running into him. Plus, by approaching him, you're being the bigger man.

Hit and run. "The average topic is exhausted in 7 to 10 minutes," says Tunnicliffe. That makes for a great time to take your leave. If you're at a party or business event, it's your duty to socialize with as many people as you can, anyway.

Avoid hot spots. He's an insufferable New York Yankees fan. (Is there any other kind?) You're a long-suffering Boston Red Sox fan. (Is there any other kind?) So what do you talk about? Anything but baseball. Steer clear of any topics that you know are going to set you at each other's throats. If he brings it up, move quickly to a different topic.

Focus on the positive. "You can always find something you like about a person," says Tunnicliffe. Ask him questions until you do. Afterwards, he'll think much more highly of you, too, for your interest in him.

Burn no bridges. Yes, he's a pompous idiot. But everybody is a potential client, a possible supervisor, or a likely ally at some point. By making the effort to be civil, you're making sure that your own future is paved smoothly.

Tell a Joke

"Ha ha ha ha ha, gasp, ha ha, hack, cough."

That's you, busting a gut after Mortimer across the hall told you one of the funniest jokes you've ever heard.

Deathly silence.

That's the reaction you get when you repeat the same joke later that day. How come? Why is your version about as funny as a loose toenail in your underwear? More than 200 years ago, famed author Jonathan Swift was lamenting the same issue. "All human race would fain be wits. And millions miss, for one that hits," he wrote.

"There is a complete art in setting up a joke," explains Jack Burditt, a comedy writer and co-executive producer for the NBC television sitcom *Just Shoot Me*. Burditt knows a thing or two about humor—he won two Emmy awards for his work on the show *Frasier* and, before that, he won a Golden Globe and a Peabody award while writing for *Mad about You*.

Being the Good Humor Man

Pulling off a rolling-in-the-aisles kind of joke demands the skills of a storyteller, says Burditt. "A good joke sucks the listener in; it brings him into the story." You want to paint a picture in the listener's mind; you want to make it real for him. Here are some points to remember.

Don't be afraid to fail. Face it, if you're not a natural at joke telling, you're going to bomb at first. "Sometimes, the best thing is to tell the joke, fail, and then figure out why you failed," says Burditt. Don't be thin-skinned about it. See yourself as a work in progress.

Adopt a watchful attitude. Go back to Mortimer and, this time, pay attention to the way he tells the joke. What makes it funny? What do you enjoy about his method? "Try to get into other people's heads," says Burditt.

Try out your material. In comedy, practice really does make perfect. The great stand-up comics practice lines and jokes incessantly, says Burditt. He and his co-writers practice lines on each other all the time. Find a willing partner, or stand in front of a mirror and watch what you're doing.

Make it relevant. People often laugh because they see themselves or someone they know in the joke, explains Burditt. Nothing says you have to repeat a joke verbatim—most jokes can be customized to make them more apropos to the particular listener or audience. For example, instead of starting off, "There was a young girl from Nantucket . . . ," you could start with, "There was a young girl from Boise . . ." if that's where you happen to be.

Develop better timing than a Swiss watchmaker. You've heard about that elusive thing known as timing. Yes, it's important. Try timing a joke differently on each attempt. Add a longer pause here, a shorter one there, especially right before the punch line. "I still don't get why a five-second pause is often 10 times as funny as a two-second pause, but that's the way it is," says Burditt.

Know your audience. If you're Dennis Rodman in Salt Lake City, nothing you say is going to be funny. Same with your jokes. If it's not appropriate humor for the situation, don't even try.

Be persistent in your quest to improve, but don't get so wound up that you, um, lose your sense of humor. Then, of course, the joke would be on you.

Twinkle, twinkle, and be a star. Bob Hope. Jack Benny. Jerry Seinfeld. Rich Little. All the top comedians have had it. It's the gleam. The mischievous twinkle in the eye that tells you something good is coming up. It makes you atwitter with anticipation. By the time the punch line arrives, you'd laugh at wet sawdust. It's like you're laughing inwardly, says Burditt, and it's infectious to those listening to you. Let the mirth show in your eyes.

Apologize

Hugh Grant got it right.

When Los Angeles police discovered the British actor receiving fellatio from a hooker in 1995, many figured that his boyish, charming, and innocent public image was, ah, blown. Some asked if his career would survive the paid affections of prostitute Divine Brown. Others speculated that his long-time girlfriend, Elizabeth Hurley, would ditch him.

Instead, after a spate of sincere public (and, most assuredly, private) apologies, the Oxford grad's career went on to new heights. The stunningly beautiful Hurley stayed with him. Grant's tomb was rent open.

How did he do it? For the answer, we went to William L. Benoit, Ph.D., professor of communication at the University of Missouri in Columbia and author of *Accounts, Excuses, and Apologies: A Theory of Image Restoration Discourse*. Besides studying Grant's success in parlaying a $60 dalliance into forgiveness, Dr. Benoit has researched many of the nation's public-relations nightmares. You, too, can use the techniques he has formulated for your own acts of contrition.

Assess the Situation

The first question you need to answer is how hot is the water you're in? Some social infractions only require a quick, heartfelt "Sorry about that." But don't kid yourself—that apology is still important. If you bump into someone in the hallway and just walk off wordless, a minor incident can turn into a grudge.

For those more serious transgressions, you need to pull out some more intensive strategies. Dr. Benoit suggests you keep in mind the following.

Accept that it's going to be tough. "We don't like to admit we're wrong," says Dr. Benoit. "Human beings naturally value their reputations. That's an appropriate way to feel, but sometimes we have to fight our feelings and make sincere apologies."

Note the word *sincere*. "If you don't think you've done anything wrong, why are you apologizing?" asks Dr. Benoit. Hollow sorrows not only won't work, they'll make the recipient even more angry.

Tell the truth. You may choose not to reveal certain things while apologizing, but never fib. If it comes to light later—as it usually does—that you lied to cover your backside, not only will that negate your apology but also it will dig you a whole new hole. "If you had just confessed and taken your lumps, you'd only be facing one problem," reminds Dr. Benoit.

Don't waffle. Say that you're sorry. Period. Don't try to make excuses for yourself. Forget about saying things like, "Yes, I had an affair, but you haven't been very attentive to me and she initiated it and the moon was full and the grass was green and, and, and. . . ." The more you water down your apology with lame justifications, the less likely anyone is to accept it.

Maintain your dignity. Remember the words of professor Henry Higgins in *Pygmalion*. "Cease this detestable boohooing instantly," he told a whining Eliza Dolittle. Likewise, you don't want to be seen as a pathetic, driveling basket case. Show sincerity, yes; but not melodramatics.

Make it right. It doesn't matter a whit how convincing your woeful regrets are if the offended people think it's just going to happen again. "If someone has wronged us, we want him to rectify the situation," explains Dr. Benoit. You need to tell those people, in detail, what steps you'll take to make sure that whatever you did won't happen again.

Give it time. Don't forget that you're dealing with a human being. No matter how sincere your apology is, it's going to take time for forgiveness to follow. Be patient, be penitent, and remember: To err is Hugh, man; to forgive, Divine.

Sound Smarter Than You Are

Eddie the plumber used to drink beer with Raymond D. Strother, a partner in Strother, Duffy, Strother, a political consulting firm in Washington, D.C. At various times in his career, Strother has given political advice to Bill Clinton, Al Gore, Gary Hart, and many, many others. He's also the vice president of the American Association of Political Consultants.

Strother recounts, "One day, Eddie said to me, 'Look, I'm not very smart, and I don't know many words. Is there anything you can recommend to me so I don't seem as dumb as I feel?' I said, 'Well, Eddie, that's easy. Do what intellectuals do.' "

So, what do intellectuals do?

"I said, 'Eddie, just tell them it's relative,'" says Strother. If you're asked for an opinion, on any topic, the answer is the same. It's relative. Eddie tried that and was awestruck.

Eddie was so awestruck, in fact, that he came back to Strother for additional advice. He really wanted to impress his boss. Strother taught him a word—viscosity. Eddie, being a plumber, was able to use a word like viscosity to describe thick things going down a drain.

"He went around trying to find ways to work the word *viscosity* into things," recalls Strother. It impressed the hell out of Eddie's boss.

The moral of this story: Sounding smarter than you are is probably much easier than you think.

All of the People, Some of the Time

Maybe you don't qualify for Mensa. Maybe you have trouble even spelling it. No matter. Here are some tips to raise your perceived IQ.

Bone up. Ray Suarez, host of National Public Radio's *Talk of the Nation*, is faced with a two-hour show, four days a week, covering a huge number of topics. Still, he always manages to sound knowledgeable, even when it's a topic that's way out of his field. How?

Homework. "The method for prep is to not try to learn everything the night before," he explains. "That would be like trying to cram for a final in a class you've never attended."

He knows what topics are likely to come up and starts scanning the papers and television for information. You can do the same. If you know you have a dinner party with the boss and his florist friends, check out some books on flower arranging. If you're going to a big bluegrass revival concert, borrow a few compact discs from the library and read the dust jackets. Again, the idea is to know a few things about the topic well enough to carry on an intelligent conversation about them.

Find an expert. When something really big happens in the world, what do the talking heads on TV do? They ask experts to tell us what it all means. You can do the same. If a big event is coming up and you know nothing about it, find someone who does, says Dr. William L. Benoit of the University of Missouri.

"You can't know everything about everything," Dr. Benoit says. Find someone who knows the score and ask him to give you a nutshell description of the important issues at hand. Odds are, he'll be flattered that you thought highly enough of him to ask his opinion.

Take your time. When someone throws you a conversational curveball, don't blurt out the first thing that pops into your head. There's no time limit on answers. And there are two hidden benefits in going slow. "One, you might think of something to say," says Dr. Benoit. "Two, people may get the impression that you're being thoughtful." Little do they know that you're trying to figure out how to scratch unobtrusively.

Hold your ground. As the host of the

popular game show *Jeopardy!*, Alex Trebek makes a living appearing smart. True, he really *is* smart, but even he estimates that he only knows about two-thirds of the material on the show. So what happens when conversations in his real life wander into the few areas where he isn't knowledgeable? One trick Trebek uses is to substitute clever humor in place of actual knowledge and steer the talk back to familiar ground. For example, if the discussion turns to the philosophical meaning of sanity, Trebek suggests saying: "I love the sanatee. I go to see them in the Florida waters all the time."

Here's another variation on the same theme. Say the bleeding heart historians start talking about Dame Edith Cavell, the noted English nurse executed by Germans in the First World War. You could casually say, "Enos Cabell? I think the Dodgers lost a great third baseman when he retired." Not only do you save face, you get to turn the talk to baseball.

"I can do stuff like this hoping that the stupid thing that I'm saying will be recognized as such by intelligent people because they know that I know better," says Trebek. Plus, unlike on *Jeopardy!*, you get extra points for creativity.

But Not All of the People All of the Time

Strother once worked on the campaign of a candidate for governor of Louisiana. "This guy was so dumb that he once bragged to me how he went all the way through law school and never once in his life finished a whole book," says Strother.

He taught his gubernatorial candidate all the tricks. The candidate even used the word "viscosity" in his television ads. He was always

---

The Sounds of Silence

Sometimes, the most intelligent thing you can say is nothing at all.

Learn to manage your silences; doing so can be much better than speaking, says Washington, D.C., political consultant Raymond D. Strother. "If you have a really dumb guy, teach him to use silence."

It's a sentiment echoed by Dr. William L. Benoit of the University of Missouri. If you're in an unfamiliar situation, he says, mum is your most useful word. "If you're talking a lot and grasping at straws, you'll say things that are contradictory," he says. "Clearly, that doesn't make you look smarter."

Replace your words with knowing nods, bemused smiles, and thoughtful glances.

---

photographed and filmed in the company of Louisiana's brightest minds: scientists, civic leaders, top businessmen. And for months, he was leading in the polls. Then, as election day neared, the politico began to drop. He ran second, then third, finally ending up last. Curious and frustrated, Strother conducted some exit polls.

"The reason my guy slipped to fourth was because people didn't think he was smart enough," recalls Strother. There's a valuable lesson to be learned here. Louisiana political campaigns run for about a year and a half. By the time voting day rolled around, people had the man figured out.

There's a statute of limitations on your smart act. Eventually, people will see through it. If you're faking intelligence, consider yourself on a dive-bombing mission. Fly in there, hit 'em with all your armament, and then get the heck out of there before they catch on.

Oh, and don't run for governor.

Answer a Child's Questions

So, what do you want to be? A perennial Mediterranean plant or a man revered for his profound wisdom? Both are definitions of the word *sage*.

If you have kids, the choice has already been made for you. You've been saved from the turkey stuffing, you profound man you. Children pummel you with their ceaseless inquiries because, to them, you *are* a sage.

"Here you have these little creatures looking up to you and asking you questions because you are the fountain of great wisdom and knowledge," says Wade F. Horn, Ph.D., president of the National Fatherhood Initiative and author of *The New Father Book: What Every New Father Needs to Know to Be a Good Dad.*

Boy, good thing they don't know that you still can't figure out how to work a self-cleaning oven. But there it is—you're the *Funk and Wagnalls* of fathering. It's a distinct honor, really. Children tend to ask questions of those they trust. Of course, they may just ply a boulder with queries when you're not around. But we owe it to them to do our best to guide them through the magical world they see all around. Remember, we tend to be a bit old and jaded, but to them, it's all fresh and new.

Answering the Stumpers

We posed some of the tougher questions that dads get hit with to the experts. Here are their answers. One general rule to keep in mind: Keep your answers appropriate to the child's age.

Daddy, what is that hairy thing? "That's just something that boys have that girls don't," suggests Alan Hawkins, Ph.D., assistant professor of family sciences at Brigham Young University in Provo, Utah, and an expert in fathering. At an early age, that should suffice. At that point, they're more interested in how people are different than in a lecture on the human reproductive tract.

Daddy, did you do drugs? This brings up a valuable point. Some things are just off-limits. "If my kid came to me and asked, 'Daddy, what positions do you and Mommy use?' I'd say that it's none of his business," says Dr. Horn. "The idea that we have to answer every one of our kids' questions just because they ask is not one that I buy into."

Instead, redirect the focus to the child. Explain to him the real dangers associated with drug use, but don't exaggerate by saying he will go to hell if he uses them or will become a heroin addict by taking a hit on a joint. Kids spot hyperbole easily, and it damages your credibility. Tell him that life is cool enough on its own and doesn't need any artificial enhancement.

Daddy, where do babies come from? Dr. Hawkins's son hit him with that one when he was five. "So, he got a 5-year-old's response. It doesn't require all the details that they get when they're 12 or 13," he says. Babies happen when a mommy and a daddy love each other very much and come together to make one. Then the baby grows in Mommy's tummy until it's ready to come out and be born. Save the birds and bees talk until puberty, Dr. Hawkins advises.

Daddy, what are you and Mommy doing? First of all, lock the door. A hook and eye costs about a buck down at the hardware store. "This happens to every parent," Dr. Horn says. Just say you were getting ready to sleep or that you were spending private time together. Above all, don't freak out and overreact.

"Overreacting communicates that you were doing something bad," says Dr. Horn. You don't want your kids to think that approaching you is treacherous stuff, or that sex is a bad thing. Calmly ask them to leave you in peace for a few minutes. This is a good time to break out the *Barney* videotapes.

Daddy, why do people die? Tough one. Tough situation, tough question. If you have a religious background, you can explain it in those terms, says Dr. Hawkins. If not, explain that people, like everything else, get sick or old or have accidents. This is one case where you're better off talking with your arms. "Chances are, they're not really dealing with it as a philosopher would," says Dr. Hawkins. "They just don't understand and they hurt." Break out your best teddy bear hug. They want to be reassured that you're still alive and there for them.

Daddy, are you and Mommy ever going to get divorced? This one comes at an age where they see other kids with divorced parents. They may even have picked up on some marital discord between the two of you. "I would hope that couples can answer positively to that and say, 'We love each other very much and never want to do that,'" says Dr. Hawkins.

At the same time, you need to explain why other parents get divorced. Sometimes, people stop loving each other and need to live apart. "Kids aren't dumb. They understand that if it happened to other parents, it can happen to theirs," adds Dr. Hawkins. What they're really looking for is reassurance. Give it to them. Even if there's a chance your marriage may be breaking up in the future, there's no point in trying to force them to come to terms with something that hasn't happened yet and may not happen.

Take a Break

It's no secret that a determined young lad or lass can pepper you with questions faster than a presidential special prosecutor. Trying to keep up can leave you with a tongue drier than a Johnny Carson joke.

What's also happening here is that the child just wants to feel connected with you. If

---

Nothing but Blue Skies

It's a question that is as much a part of childhood as skinned knees and first kisses. Why is the sky blue, Daddy?

Wouldn't it be nice to be able to answer that? Well, now you can, thanks to David F. Young, a senior research scientist at NASA's Langley Research Center in Hampton, Virginia, and an atmospheric whiz. Here's Young's explanation.

The technical term for the cause is Rayleigh scattering. Think of it in terms of a prism. You know how when sunlight goes through a prism, it gets broken down into its individual colors? Similar principle here. Except the sunlight is broken down in the atmosphere by gas molecules such as oxygen and nitrogen.

These molecules are so tiny that they bend the smallest wavelengths of light—the blues—the most. And there are kazillions of them, so they scatter the blue light all over the sky. A funny thing about Rayleigh scattering is that it can also cause parts of the sky to be other colors than blue. You can prove this for yourself.

On the next sunny day, stand with either shoulder to the sun and look straight ahead. This is where the sky is the deepest blue. Now take a peek in the direction of the sun (remember, don't stare directly into it). You'll see that the sky near the sun is actually a pale yellow. This is because the blue light is scattered away from your line of sight, and you get what's left over.

This effect is even stronger at sunset when so much blue is removed that the sky turns yellow and red, Young explains.

---

your mouth needs a rest, use your arms. Sweep the kid up in a playful hug and engage him in something more physical.

That should buy you about 10 seconds.

Deliver a Eulogy

And now, for something completely different . . .

When Monty Python member Graham Chapman died in 1989, fellow trouper John Cleese was one of the eulogists. "I said, good riddance to bad rubbish, that he was a lazy, drunken old freeloader, and we were better off without him," Cleese recalled in an interview with the *Washington Post.*

After a moment's pause, the mourners burst into laughter.

Granted, you would expect irreverent humor at any gathering of the manic British comedy troupe, even a funeral. But there is an important lesson here for all of us: Joyful remembering helps heal and also is a fitting celebration of a life.

"Sometimes a well-timed laugh is so important," says the Reverend Father Richard B. Gilbert, executive director of the World Pastoral Care Center in Valparaiso, Indiana, and author of *Heartpeace: Healing Help for Grieving Folks.* He also offers extensive programs and support services on bereavement, pastoral care, and spirituality.

A Life Remembered

How do you sum up someone's life in mere words? How do you, in a single offering, capture everything that you and the others around you held dear in the person who died?

Well, you can't, and you shouldn't feel you need to try. A simple eulogy cannot entirely represent the magic that was a human being's life. But it can play an invaluable part in helping you and others start on the path to dealing with your grief.

"Eulogies are a small piece of a much larger picture, that of healthy grieving," says Reverend Gilbert, who has conducted hundreds of funerals. He offers this advice when giving a eulogy.

Talk it out. While your eulogy is very much your personal remembrances and thoughts, you don't need to be a one-man show. Sit down with friends and family and talk about it. Reverend Gilbert did this while working on his own father's eulogy. "We laughed and we cried. Then we picked out two or three things and shared them."

Write it down. A written eulogy not only keeps you steady while delivering it, but writing in itself has advantages. "Writing is very therapeutic," says Reverend Gilbert. It's a way of dealing with some very convoluted emotions, even if you decide not to share everything.

Give thanks and ask for help. Thank the people who supported the family during their time of grief. And ask them to continue. Days, weeks, and months from now, you'll still need friends to turn to, shoulders to cry on.

Avoid loaded issues. Let's face it. Sometimes the person who died was not a model citizen. You may have a lot of unresolved emotions around that. Be honest in what you remember, but the negative stuff can be dealt with later. "You can't put all the weight on the funeral," explains Reverend Gilbert.

Go to the pros. Sometimes, after even your best efforts, you're just plain stumped. Ask for help from the funeral director. He's a trained professional in many aspects of grief. "The funeral director is not just a businessman," notes Reverend Gilbert. "He is there to provide care and service and support." That includes eulogies.

Be yourself. You aren't expected to be perfect. Speak slowly and clearly. If you choke up, take a few minutes to compose yourself. If you can't go on, people will understand. Have copies of your eulogy available at the exits so that your thoughts can go home with them. "The power of just being up there is very important," Reverend Gilbert says.

Part Eight

Real-Life Scenarios

Quest for the Best

They are modern-day Renaissance men, deftly balancing highly successful careers with fascinating and varied interests. Just when you think you have them pegged, they move off in a new and surprising direction. So can you.

You Can Do It!

These guys work hard, just like you. They also have figured out how to make time in their busy lives for the things they love. You can too.

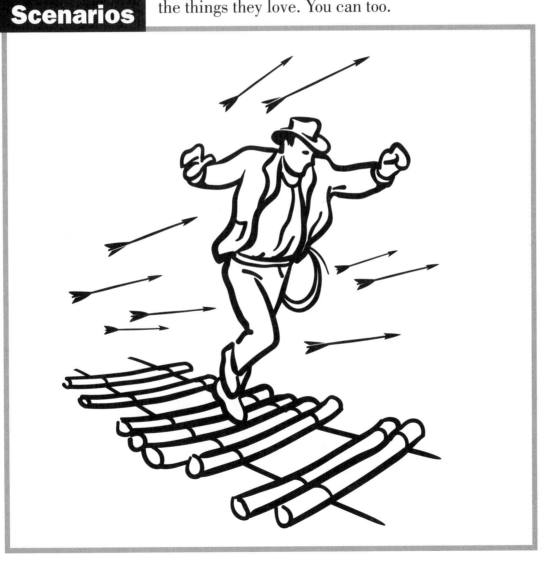

Quest for the Best

They are modern-day Renaissance men, deftly balancing highly successful careers with fascinating and varied interests. Just when you think you have them pegged, they move off in a new and surprising direction. So can you.

Tim Green, Author and Ex-Football Player

A Life in Balance

Perhaps nobody better defies the stereotype of "dumb jock" than Tim Green. Sure, he was a great athlete: All-American at Syracuse University in New York, where he was co-captain of the team his senior year. First-round 1986 draft pick (17th overall) of the Atlanta Falcons, for whom he played eight seasons, mostly as a defensive end.

But Green's talents aren't limited to pummeling beefy offensive linemen and sacking slippery quarterbacks. This is a guy who was a Rhodes scholar nominee and co-valedictorian at Syracuse (with a 3.83 grade point average in English literature), has a law degree, works as a commentator for National Public Radio and Fox's NFL game coverage, and has written four novels and two nonfiction books.

"I was kind of stuck in a football player's body, but I always wanted to write," Green says. "My teammates were never disparaging toward my intellectual bent. And I was never condescending about it. I never tried to hold myself forth as being more or less important than anybody else on my team. I just happened to read books and write books."

It's not as if the 250-

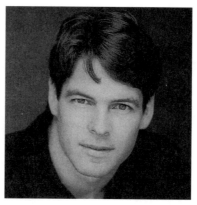

pound Green was a nerd. "I'd go and drink beers with the guys and stay out late and go golfing or bowling or whatever we were doing. But on the plane and in the locker room, instead of playing cards or goofing around, I would read. The guys were great about it. There is such a diversity of characters in the NFL. People get this stereotype, and it's shallow."

Green spent the off-seasons during his NFL career earning a law degree from Syracuse. Although he is a member of the New York State Bar Association, he doesn't actively practice law. Hard as it may be for most of us to imagine, Green viewed law school as almost a fallback career.

"I joined a firm when I first graduated," he says. "There are just so many other things that have happened that I wasn't able to keep doing it. I went to law school because I didn't know if I'd be able to broadcast games or make a living as a writer when I finished playing, and I didn't want to get to the end of my football career and just have my four-year English degree."

A Novel Approach to Football

The first book Green had published was a memoir, *The Dark Side of the Game: My Life in the NFL.* The series of essays on subjects ranging from Green's 12 concussions to drug use by players to the sport's connections to the mob made a smashing debut, becoming a

New York Times bestseller. Its success enabled Green to snag a three-book contract with Warner Books.

Each of Green's novels is a thriller with an NFL backdrop. In *The Red Zone*, a star linebacker named Luther Zorn tries to prove his innocence of the murder of the team's owner—whose wife was having an affair with the player. He makes no apologies for the recurring football themes. "My plan is to become a franchise novelist so people identify with my books and the type of books they are," he says. "I think you need that consistency. Besides, the NFL is such a great world to set stories in. There's a lot of money; there's violence and greed and corruption and drugs and treachery and jealousy. It's a rich, rich world."

There is one downside to writing football-themed thrillers, according to Green. "I think that, before they've read my books, a lot of people think, 'Oh, come on, a football player, you can't write.' They don't know I was an English major, I studied creative writing, I'm a lawyer. I think that's a stereotype that I definitely have to overcome. I haven't helped myself in that regard by choosing to set my stories in the world of football."

Green says writing novels is easier and more satisfying than writing nonfiction. "*Dark Side* was more laborious," he says. His other nonfiction book, *A Man and His Mother: One Man's Search for His Biological Mother and an Understanding of His Adoptive Mother*, was even tougher.

That book details Green's search for his birth mother. "That was tough to write," recalls Green, who is adopted. "I turned myself inside out for that book. It was very cathartic."

Trouble was, Green's editor and his agent hated the first draft of the book. It was even suggested that somebody else write it for him. "It was a tremendous insult," he says. But he had to admit that the critiques had merit. "A lot of it was self-indulgent. It was bad."

Green insisted on constructive criticism rather than letting somebody else write his story. He even offered to return his advance if the book wasn't published. And so he plugged away at the revised version. "Everybody was thrilled with the second draft," he says.

By the way, Green did find his birth mother, who lives in Boston. They speak once or twice a week.

Now Green is back to crafting the sort of novels he likes to read. "I like to be entertained when I read," he says. "I like a book that's fast-paced with good characters—where you pick it up and it starts fast and a day or so later you stay up late because you have to finish it."

Working and Workouts

While writing keeps Green busy, the father of four makes spending time with his family a priority. "The good thing about what I do is I can do it from home," he says. Home is on a lake in upstate New York. Many summer days find Green water-skiing and snorkeling with his family.

Green was blessed with looks, athleticism, and brains, but he attributes his success to two other traits. "One, I try to be really efficient with my time," he says. He cites as an example his daily workouts at home.

"While I work out, I'm either on the phone—I have a headset—or during football season, I have a lot of videotape that I have to watch for my job at Fox, so I'm watching tape while I'm working out.

"Second, I learned a relentlessness from the game of football, or maybe that was why I was able to succeed in football. You get pummeled and knocked down every day, and you learn to be resilient. So if someone says, 'This manuscript is no good,' you don't fold up. You don't say, 'I'm no good.' You just keep going. I've gotten knocked down in everything I've tried to do, from writing to television.

"I think the key is perseverance. You can't learn it more clearly than you do in the game of football."

Bruce Wayne, Millionaire and Socialite

A Gotham City Giant

Bruce Wayne has traveled all around the world. And though the millionaire playboy could have spent his days lounging in chateaus and villas and island retreats scattered about the globe, his jet-setting ways actually began as an early quest for knowledge—and perhaps the chance to escape a painful past.

"In my early teens, I sort of struck out on my own," Wayne recalls. "I must have attended 50 colleges, universities, and trade schools over the next five years. One professor said I seemed to have very narrow interests—I often mastered only a single aspect of a subject, and then I'd dash off to somewhere else, often in a different country."

But no matter where he traveled, Wayne says he couldn't wait to return to the gritty, urban reality of Gotham City. "The Waynes have deep roots in Gotham, going back at least 200 years, and one should honor one's ancestors, I believe. Actually, I'm quite comfortable here and never quite at home anywhere else. When I'm traveling, I always feel a bit like a bat out of hell, if you'll pardon a small, but quite clever, joke," he says, smiling a strangely sinister smile.

The response is "vintage Bruce," according to the social-page editors and the executives who run the millionaire's numerous businesses and philanthropic organizations. But sources closer to Wayne say that the millionaire's devotion to Gotham City, both in business and personal life, borders on obsessive. That his laissez-faire attitude is a veneer, a mask. They believe that under that cowl of superficiality lies a noble man who has risen above great personal tragedy to be-

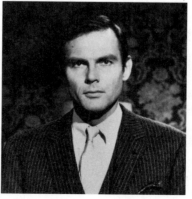

come a defender of the weak, a man who has used his vast family wealth to become a champion of the oppressed. Gotham City, it appears, has more than one crusader.

But for a tragic twist of fate, Bruce Wayne's life might have been as idle and carefree as outsiders seem to think it is.

"I suppose I did have a privileged childhood—at least until I was eight. Then I lost both my parents," he says, unwilling to discuss the matter further. And who can blame him? On a dark night, on their way home from a movie in Gotham's fashionable Park Row, Dr. Thomas and Mrs. Martha Wayne were brutally shot to death by a small-time mugger. Young Bruce watched it happen.

For a time, the orphaned Wayne was raised by the family butler, Alfred Pennyworth (who still serves Wayne to this day). Little else is known about Wayne's life until his teens, when he began his jet-setting, university-hopping ways. The young dilettante would be gone from his beloved Gotham for years.

A Prodigal Son

When Wayne finally returned, the once-proud city had declined in his absence. Even upscale Park Row, the neighborhood where Wayne lost his parents, had become known as Crime Alley. Indeed, it seemed the entire city had been given over to a criminal element, both on the street and in the highest offices of Gotham City's government and police force. "I'm actually quite concerned about crime," Wayne insists. "My butler, Alfred, listens to the radio news, and some of the stories he relays to me make me shiver."

He reopened the ancestral home, stately Wayne manor, a scant 14 miles outside of Gotham. Then, Bruce Wayne set out to save Gotham City—the only way he knew how. The young millionaire began infusing money into Gotham's ailing economy. He parlayed his family fortune into a series of increasingly daring and lucrative business ventures, all locally based.

Meanwhile, among his contacts in Gotham's social and political elite, Wayne was known for his early and outspoken support of police captain James Gordon, who would eventually rise to the office of commissioner, eradicating graft and corruption in Gotham's law enforcement community as he went.

More quietly, Wayne also began to create and fund nonprofit organizations like the Wayne Foundation and the Victims' Incorporated Program, devoted to helping crime victims and the disadvantaged of Gotham. Some years ago, Wayne personally adopted and saw to the upbringing of a young boy named Dick Grayson, who, like Wayne, was orphaned when criminals murdered his parents (the famed circus aerialists known as the Flying Graysons). Some insiders say that Wayne's obsession with spending so much of his money helping others is derived from some misplaced guilt over his parents' deaths. Meanwhile, more than a few financial wags have said Wayne is just a savvy businessman who knows a good tax break when he sees it.

His Darkest Secret?

Whatever his motivations, the Wayne presence in Gotham has made a difference. Local industry and the economy have enjoyed their longest period of prosperity in the city's 200-plus year history. And crime has dropped exponentially, although anyone familiar with Gotham City knows that has more to do with the legends and sightings of the mysterious Caped Crusaders Batman and Robin than with millionaire Bruce Wayne.

Or does it?

While we have no proof to back it up, for years a persistent rumor has been circulating in certain parts of Gotham society. It's not lost on some people that Bruce Wayne's return to Gotham coincided with the first sightings of the Batman a few months later. It's also interesting to note that Batman's legendary arsenal of equipment—stealth jets, helicopters, boats, cars, a utility belt filled with highly sophisticated, technologically advanced tools—would be unavailable to a common street vigilante. You'd have to have access to a high-tech company that could funnel you their latest equipment prototypes, to say nothing of a vast amount of wealth, to acquire and maintain this equipment.

We asked Bruce Wayne, straight out: Is he secretly bankrolling Batman?

Instantly, the playboy's bored expression is gone, replaced by a genuine grin and a powerful laugh.

"Ask me if I'm bankrolling the Loch Ness monster or the Abominable Snowman," he says, shaking his head. Then, he turns serious. "My opinion of this Batman is that he's just an urban myth, and not a very amusing one, at that."

He smiles, adding, "I much prefer Superman—the red cape really makes a statement."

Ultimately, making a statement is just as important to Wayne as anything else he does. Whether in business or charity, Wayne wants to make that all-important impression. It's evident even in his final words, when asked to impart some bit of his accumulated knowledge to our readers.

"I'm told that mutual funds and tax-free municipal bonds are a good place to put money, though I really couldn't say," he replies. "But I feel very powerfully that I can offer a guiding principle that will serve anyone who heeds it quite well: Never—and I mean never, with no exceptions—wear brown shoes after six."

We suspect that when Bruce Wayne goes out into Gotham's dark night, the only thing he wears . . . is black.

Special thanks to Dennis O'Neil, group editor at DC Comics in New York, for his invaluable help in securing this interview.

Alex Trebek,
Jeopardy! Host

In the Form of a Question

The category is famous men. For a Daily Double, this is the man who leads the number one quiz show in America. This is the man who is synonymous with knowledge. This is the man who is one of the most popular faces on television.

Too easy. Who is Alex Trebek?

But if you peer behind the little blue Daily Double screen, you will discover a man who is as at home with a hammer as he is entertaining some of Hollywood's top names. A man who is a devoted father. A man who can sip the finest wine on one day and play down-and-dirty recreational hockey the next. A man who exudes intelligence and refinement, yet remains a regular guy.

Perhaps it can be traced to his roots. Long before his days of fame, Trebek grew up in Sudbury, a hardscrabble mining town in northern Ontario. It's a place where, if you look down, the scraped rocks are blackened with mine soot and dried sweat. A place where, if you look up, the blue sky seems to stretch forever and the northern lights whisper at night.

Perhaps it was in Sudbury that Trebek learned that a man must keep his eyes skyward to see where he is headed, but his feet must be skilled enough to pick a path through life's rough terrain.

Trebek first ended up in front of American television cameras as the host of the game show *The Wizard of Odds*. His solid on-camera presence and quick wit soon had other shows knocking on his door. In 1984, it was *Jeopardy!* that knocked the loudest. In less time than he allows for Final Jeopardy, Trebek was a household name.

The demands of the show are huge. Each year, Trebek scours North America with the scouting team—looking for the brightest, most interesting contestants. The show also broadcasts from remote locations on a regular basis. Trebek even makes special trips to U.S. military bases around the world to audition the men and women in uniform.

And even after the *Jeopardy!* time clock has been punched, he's not done. In his limited spare time, he works with a number of charities and educational outfits. He's the host of the annual National Geography Bee and a board member of the National Geographic Society Education Foundation. He also serves on the board of the National Advisory Council for the Literary Volunteers of America and is very involved with the World Vision charitable organization.

Working with charities is selfish stuff, admits Trebek. Selfish in that it exposes him to incredible people. "Even though there are problems that exist in our society, there are thousands and even millions who have overcome those problems and are able to shine," he says. Being caught up in that shine is a pretty amazing place to be, adds Trebek.

The Road to the Top

Trebek left Sudbury to attend the University of Ottawa. After graduating, he began work as a journalist for the Canadian Broadcasting Corporation. While at CBC, Trebek covered national news and special events for both the television and radio divisions.

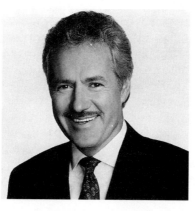

Life Off Camera

Trebek walks between two worlds. And he does it well.

He holds degrees in philosophy. He is passionate about wine and even owns his own vineyard, which bottles under the Creston label. He speaks French fluently. He owns a thoroughbred horse farm just outside of Paso Robles in central California. He golfs at exotic courses worldwide. He entertains some of Hollywood's top names in his Studio City, California, home.

But his philosophies are not airy, ethereal musings. He holds philosophy up to one standard: Does it work in real life? "Anything you learn, you should try hard to find some way to apply it to your daily existence," he says.

And the house that he wines and dines in? He helped build it. "I was there hammering and wallboarding." Now, when he sits back and waxes philosophic on the benefits of constructing one's own home, he can find the pipe when it springs a leak. As for the wining and dining, as often as not, you'll find him in the kitchen doing the cooking.

It seems only appropriate that one of Trebek's personal heroes is Mark Twain. Trebek, like Twain, considers a paintbrush as mighty as a pen.

Fatherhood—No Trivial Pursuit

Trebek became a father late in life. He was 51 when his first child, Matthew Alexander, was born in 1991. He and his wife, Jean, also have a daughter, Emily Grace. His children are the apples of his eye. Go ahead, ask him what he adores most about fatherhood.

"Oh, I don't know," he reflects. "The added responsibility, the fear, the trying to control your anger." Add to that the escalating expense of rearing children, the heart-wrenching moments when they take a tumble, the uncertainty over what kind of world we're leaving them, and a man might start to wonder why he got into this predicament in the first place. Not Trebek. He understands fully why men become fathers.

"Because we're stupid. We want unconditional love from somebody. Of course, that's also why we buy dogs."

Meet the humorous side of Trebek. Never one to resist a wisecrack, he also rarely misses the humor in a moment, even if it's at his own expense. "I love laughing at myself," he says. "I do some pretty silly things sometimes, so there's lots of material there."

Seriously though, folks, Trebek has two words of advice for other men considering becoming fathers. "Try it," he says. Nowhere else will you find the joys, the magic, the love that comes with being a dad. Plus, you'll have a captive audience for your jokes.

Trebek on Knowledge

The acquisition of knowledge is something that has served Trebek well, both in his professional and personal lives. You might think that, being swamped all day with questions and answers, he might get a bit gun-shy of anything even slightly resembling new information. Not so.

"I love learning," he says. With a bit of extra time, he would unhesitatingly enroll in university again. He looks for knowledge in things as simple as purchasing some furniture. How it's made, where it comes from, who created its style. "And why it costs so damn much," he quips. Learning, indeed, is an everyday experience.

So how, with this love of knowledge, would he do as a contestant on *Jeopardy!?* "If I were in the seniors tournament, I would probably do very well," he says. "In the regular game, where the contestants are faster, it would be tough for me."

Trebek figures that, without the answer—or is that question?—cards in front of him, he would know about two-thirds of the correct responses. Nothing to sneeze at. See if you can get that many right the next time you watch the show.

If you can, let him know the next time you pass his driveway. Chances are good that you'll catch him underneath a red 1971 Italia convertible he's restoring.

Bring with you three things—your wit, your wrench, and your Wittgenstein.

Henry Winkler, Actor, Director, and Producer

Happy Days Are Here Again

At one time, Henry Winkler wasn't concentrating on being a well-rounded, worldly, successful man—he was just trying to make it through the next day. Now, Winkler, who took the television world by storm as the ultracool Arthur Fonzarelli on the hit show *Happy Days*, is recognized almost everywhere in the world. But it wasn't always this way.

Growing up with undiagnosed dyslexia, Winkler was not only at the bottom of his high school class but also was ranked in the lowest 3 percent of the country's students. His written language skills were atrocious and his math abilities were nearly nonexistent due to his inability to comprehend textbooks. He was branded as lazy, not living up to his potential. Slowly, surely, over the course of many years, his self-image fell to the level of his tenuous trigonometry marks.

How does a man shake off such a debilitating condition and not only go on to succeed, but to excel in ways that most people only dream of?

"It was hard," he recalls. "There are times when you actually think, 'Oh my God, I have no idea what I'm doing. Everybody is telling me I'm stupid or lazy.'" And yet, despite his serious self-doubts, he knew that if he kept his eyes on where he wanted to go, eventually he'd find a way to get there.

"I always knew what I wanted, and I always felt I could somehow get it," he says. How that would happen, he decided, would take care of itself. His job was to just keep going.

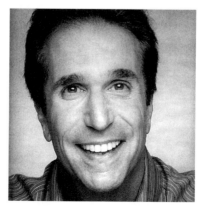

"There is something inside you that keeps moving forward," he explains. "You must never lose sight of what you want."

One of his first decisions along that path was to continue in school, regardless of the miserable years spent in high school. Winkler left his native New York City for Emerson College in Boston, majoring in drama and also studying child psychology. He later went on to the Yale School of Drama, where he was awarded a master of fine arts degree.

After a short stint with the Yale Repertory Company, Winkler made his way back to New York. To put bread on the table and build up his list of credits, he churned out dozens of radio and television commercials. He toured briefly with a children's theater troupe, starred in an ill-fated Broadway production, and managed to break into feature films. He and the then-unknown Sylvester Stallone co-starred as leather-jacketed thugs in *The Lords of Flatbush*.

Winkler's second feature film, *Crazy Joe*, took him to Hollywood. After a few guest appearances on *The Mary Tyler Moore Show*, *The Bob Newhart Show*, and *Rhoda*, Winkler's years of reaching for the stars finally made him a star.

The Fonz Is Born

On October 30, 1973, his twenty-eighth birthday, Henry Winkler was cast as Arthur Fonzarelli. *Happy Days'* producers never intended for the Fonz to be the star of the show. But soon, audiences at *Happy Days* shootings were going berserk whenever the Fonz sauntered through the Cunninghams' kitchen door. Kids were flipping their thumbs in the air, and "Ayyyy!" and "Whooa!" became part of the American lexicon.

The rest is a piece of television folklore. The Fonz's leather jacket now hangs in the

Smithsonian. And a whole new generation of kids is finding the Fonz and company, as *Happy Days* plays in reruns as one of the most-watched shows in Nickelodeon's Nick at Nite lineup.

Meanwhile, Winkler is not resting on his laurels. After *Happy Days* drew to a close in 1984, he found himself reluctant to continue in acting. "I don't know if it was fear at the idea of not being able to duplicate the success of the Fonz, or just sheer exhaustion," he says.

And so he turned his attention to directing and producing. His film directing credits include *Memories of Me* with Billy Crystal and JoBeth Williams, and *Cop and a Half* with Burt Reynolds. His production efforts have rewarded him equally well with the success of movies like *The Sure Thing* and *Young Sherlock Holmes*.

Early on in his wildly successful career as the Fonz, Winkler had concerns about being typecast—anathema to the idea of being well-rounded. Some of that concern came from the people around him warning him of that possibility, some from his own ideas of where he would like his life to go.

"It's almost as if my parents named me Henry 'Fonzie' Winkler," he says in a tip of the hat to the role with which most people still identify him. But—and this is a big but—he eventually realized that strength in any one field or role does not have to preclude a person from others. Actually, it's just the opposite.

"The fact is, when you look back, there are more pros than cons in what I have been able to experience in my life," he says. "The Fonz gave me much more than he took away from my life."

The household name that the character created opened many other professional and personal doors for Winkler, including the ability to travel extensively, meet fascinating people at the forefront of their fields, and spend a considerable amount of time working with children's charities, a cause that remains close to his heart. His work with children has brought him not only tremendous personal satisfaction but also recognitions such as B'nai B'rith's Champion of Youth award and a United Nations Peace Prize. Winkler and his wife, Stacey, have three children, Max, Zoe, and Jed.

Being good at what you do in one field and translating that into increased opportunities in other fields holds true for anyone, he adds. "All of a sudden, you see that there's no trick to life," he says. "It's just a matter of knowing what you want and actually living it."

A Family Man

In this journey called life and in the quest to become fulfilled, satisfied human beings, Winkler recommends a few essential traits to aid you along the way: a sense of humor, a sense of decency, and a sense of respect. "We need to think in terms of the idea that we're all in this together, that we're a community," he says. In his life and work, he puts it like this: "I only believe in ensemble. I believe totally in a group effort. I love the sense of family that is created with that."

Humor, Winkler maintains, allows the suffocating self-seriousness of life to be gently dispelled and opens the eyes to greater wonders. And, he adds, it's a key in raising children. At least some of the time. "Once in a while, I can actually make my children laugh, but most of the time, I'm either a goofball or a dork," he muses.

The urge to grow is one that virtually all people have, adds Winkler. And it need not be huge, earth-shattering growth to fuel a satisfied life. In fact, it rarely is, he says.

"Reaching beyond your grasp can be done in millimeters. We're not talking miles, yards, or even inches. It can be millimeters," he explains. The result is the same—a slow, inexorable march toward realizing your innermost dreams and becoming as well-rounded as you want to be. An added bonus: "The feeling you get from having reached in the first place is indescribable."

Clive Cussler, Author and Adventurer

The Never-Ending Search for New Horizons

What happens when you decide to live outside the lines? When your days are a series of adventures, one toppling onto the other? When intrigue, suspense, and daring are as much a part of your life as your rakish grin and your appreciation of a cold beer? Well, you could become Dirk Pitt, a fictional devil-may-care hero enjoyed by millions of readers around the world.

Or you could be his creator.

For pretty much all of his life, Clive Cussler has been mirroring fantasy with reality. And for half of that time, it's been a very lucrative endeavor. He's the author of 14 consecutive *New York Times* bestsellers and has 90 million books in print, virtually all starring the man with the mesmeric opaline green eyes, Dirk Pitt. From his first bestseller, *Raise the Titanic*, to the latest, *Flood Tide*, Cussler has brought his love of adventure to the world.

Okay, so that's his day job. What does he do for fun? Skiing, jogging, swimming, hiking, cycling, and diving. Plus, he's also a car-collector extraordinaire. In a garage near Golden, Colorado, he stores more than 80 models of classic and antique cars—the same ones Dirk Pitt's ladies swoon over.

There's more. A good chunk of Cussler's remaining time is spent hunting historically significant shipwrecks. Cussler, an international authority on shipwrecks, is the founder of the nonprofit National Underwater and Marine Agency (NUMA), named after the fictional outfit that Dirk Pitt works for.

Since its creation, NUMA and its troupe of volunteers and

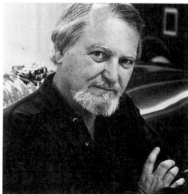

marine experts have discovered more than 60 wrecks. One of Cussler's greatest finds was the Confederate submarine *Hunley*, the first submarine to sink a ship in battle. He also located the Union *Housatonic*, the ship that was on the receiving end of *Hunley's* claim to fame.

Cussler funds most of NUMA's work through his book royalties. All artifacts are donated to museums and naval institutes. Cussler's only nonfiction book, *The Sea Hunters*, details the story behind each craft's sinking and subsequent discovery. The book was considered in lieu of a Ph.D. thesis by the State University of New York's Maritime College, which awarded Cussler a Doctor of Letters degree in 1997.

Plainly put, the guy is a modern-day Renaissance man. And what makes this even more astonishing is that he's a writer. Often, when Cussler is around other fiction writers, he'll inquire as to their pursuits outside of writing. Most of them look at him like he's a three-headed squid, maybe one that has been lurking in one of the wrecks he's found. They can't believe there are other activities beyond writing, promoting their books, arguing with editors, and demanding better deals from their agents.

"I guess so many authors are wrapped up in their work," he says wryly. "It's one thing to say you've made a lot of money, but there are other things in life."

Perhaps that would ring hollow if he had only discovered a bent for adventure after the success of his books. But the Dirk Pitt in him has always been there. Even before the big bucks.

Boxcars, Bandstands, and Bushes

In 1950, Cussler and a friend hopped in a 1939 Ford convertible and headed out across the country. They slept in boxcars, bandstands, and even in bushes next to the Capitol building in Washington, D.C. "That just wasn't done in those days," he says of the trip. "Our classmates couldn't believe anybody would just take off like that."

The lesson? Adventure can come cheap. The whole trip cost him $350.

He returned home and enlisted in the Air Force at the beginning of the hostilities in Korea. A training sergeant found out about his penchant for hot rods, and Cussler ended up in Hawaii after he completed aircraft engine school. When he wasn't working on Stratocruiser engines, he and two buddies, Al Giordano and Dave Anderson, were plying the Hawaiian waters in early diving gear, well before recreational diving was popular. Giordano became Al Giordino, Dirk Pitt's fictional sidekick.

After leaving the Air Force, he and another friend bought a gas station outside Los Angeles. Weekends were spent in a chopped-up 1948 Mercury, scouting the surrounding areas for old ghost towns, abandoned gold mines, and Spanish artifacts. "If it was lost, I looked for it," he says. Failure to find something did not equate to a fruitless day—any frustrations dealt by the unyielding earth were exorcised by shooting antique rifles at rocks in the distance.

After the gas station gig, Cussler went into advertising, ending up as creative director at two of the country's leading agencies. One of his successes was the creation of the Ajax White Knight advertising campaign.

Despite making a handsome salary for the 1960s, Cussler knew he wanted to do more. In 1965, he began writing in the evenings and on weekends. In 1973, he made a modest $5,000 from *The Mediterranean Caper*. In 1976, his breakthrough book, *Raise the Titanic*, was published and catapulted him into the realm of the highest-paid writers.

"People would say to me, 'Congratulations on your overnight success,'" he laughs. "Yeah, it only took 11 years."

Stirring the Embers

So, what's his secret? How does a man go through life doing and experiencing things that most people only dream of, making a boatload of money along the way? The secret is, there is no secret.

"You have to have a fairly active imagination to let a sense of adventure into your life," Cussler says. He believes that all people have this capability, though the Muse fires may have dimmed—it's just a matter of stoking the glowing coals. "It just lies dormant. People have fallen into routines," he says.

"Anything can be an adventure if it just takes you beyond your normal routine," he continues. "You have to be one of these people who has one eye on his family and work, but the other eye is looking over the horizon."

Through all of his adventures, Cussler has steadfastly kept one eye on his family. He has been married to Barbara Knight for more than 40 years, and the couple has three children and two grandchildren.

The key to balancing family, work, and adventure doesn't lie in the imagination, says Cussler. "Perseverance is vital," he says. "It heads the list. So many people give up too easily."

The result is another evening in front of the tube, another adventure left in the wilds. You don't have to bike over the Rockies at age 50 like Cussler did. Or take the stick of a glider at 55. Or bungee jump in British Columbia at 60. By the way, he's planning to skydive at 70.

Adventure can be climbing that hill that sits outside your backyard, he says. Or traveling to the next county to see about that postage stamp for your collection. Or using the library to find out about local sites that may yield interesting archaeological discoveries. "It's all around you," says Cussler. "The big thing is just kicking yourself off the couch and doing it. It's there."

You Can Do It! These guys work hard, just like you. They also have figured out how to make time in their busy lives for the things they love. You can too.

Communicating in the Key of Life

Rodney Moag, Ph.D., Austin, Texas

Date of birth: October 15, 1936

Profession: University language professor and country music performer/disc jockey

The title cut from my latest compact disc pretty much sums things up. I'm the "Pickin', Singin' Professor." By day, I am a tenured associate professor of South Asian language at the University of Texas in Austin, where I teach Malayalam, a language spoken in South India. At night, I perform locally and throughout central Texas with my band, Texas à la Moag. It's a gender-balanced band that plays classic country, Western swing, rockabilly, blues, and bluegrass.

Communication is the unifying theme of teaching and performing. Language is a golden key that gives you access to people that you couldn't otherwise reach. A musical performance is very interactive: You are reaching out to the audience. I love radio, both ham radio, where I talk to people, and broadcasting. I host *The Country, Swing, and Rockabilly Jamboree* and co-host *Strictly Bluegrass* on KOOP, a non-commercial community radio station in Austin. This is especially challenging because you're reaching out to people who aren't physically there, and you are programming to an audience that you can only imagine.

I started out at Syracuse University in New York in 1957, studying broadcasting, but I found myself attracted more to foreign languages. After studying Italian, Spanish, Portuguese, German, and a little Russian, I wanted to do something different, so I took up the languages of India. India was not only accessible, but there were several lifetimes of learning to be had there.

Studying and working in India was a life-changing event. Up to that time, I had nixed the idea of a teaching career. But the year I spent teaching English at the University of Patna changed my mind. Before coming to Austin, I taught at the Universities of Missouri and Michigan, and I spent three years as visiting Fulbright professor in the Fiji Islands.

When I was 11, I got my first guitar and won my first contest two months later. Subsequently, I took up mandolin, fiddle, and other instruments. Musically, 1995 was a really good year for me. I placed first in the Yodeling Contest at the Texas Heritage Music Festival, and my radio show was recognized in the *Austin Chronicle*'s "Best of Austin" media category. I was voted "Human Being of the Year" twice in a contest run by a local magazine. The magazine doesn't hold the contest anymore, so I was the final, if dubious, Human Being of the Year. It's hard to know what your competition is in a contest like that. I got into *Who's Who in America* in 1997 and 1998. I don't know how. I think they were hoping I would buy the book.

After my CD came out, a writer from a local paper asked me how I managed performances at night and teaching during the day. My secret: I try to take a nap in between. It takes high energy to carry off either a successful classroom or a club performance. The best way I've found to keep my strength up is biscuits and gravy, a chicken-fried steak, or a good plate of enchiladas now and then.

Balancing Two Lives

Gary Skoloff,
West Orange, New Jersey

Date of birth: August 9, 1933

Profession: Attorney and organic farmer

Essentially, I have two lives—two great lives. Monday through Thursday, I'm dressed in a suit and tie, practicing law at one of the largest family-law firms in New Jersey. By Friday, I'm getting dirty in rural northeastern Pennsylvania—making what we organic farmers call black gold out of my compost piles. Sometimes, I escape all my responsibilities and disappear to a World War II memorabilia show or "take to the hills" in my military jeep.

My family-law specialty led me to work on the internationally famous Baby M trial. I represented the father who was battling to retain custody of his child after the surrogate mother he hired wanted the baby back. The case is now one of the leading legal precedents concerning surrogate motherhood. I have lectured throughout the country for the American Bar Association, I teach at a local university, and I have written a three-volume book on family law.

Farm life is perfect therapy for a busy lawyer from the suburbs of West Orange, New Jersey. Some trials have gotten me into heated discussions on television. At the farm, I live in a log cabin with no television. Rather than listen to people's conflicts all day, I listen to the wind while I'm unloading hay or weeding the garden. Often at work I have to eat on the run; at the farm I go outside and pick my lunch.

At one time, it would have seemed comical: the idea of me, a New Jersey lawyer, owning a 200-acre farm, raising organic vegetables, chickens, cattle, horses, and fruit trees, and even making my own maple syrup. I'll admit that I was raised a true city boy from Newark who didn't know a broccoli plant from a weed. My wife, Shary, and I impulsively

bought the whole farm when we were just looking for a little land to camp on with our infant daughter.

Every year, we grew a few more vegetables at our "campsite," and gradually we added farm equipment, barns, and animals. Shary and I read all we could about agriculture, but mostly we learned through trial and error. It's an ongoing experiment—there's a certain cornfield where we're still raising a great bumper crop of weeds. But all in all, our harvests are successful enough to supply eggs and produce to health food stores and a bakery. We also market our vegetables, flowers, and maple syrup at a country stand from the house.

Despite their suburban existence, my daughters, Karen and Lesley, got to experience all the creative things growing up that life in the country offers. I will always cherish watching them feeding the animals, riding horses, making ice cream, clearing trails, pulling carrots out of the earth, gathering eggs, and building secret hideaways in the woods. There was so much to do with our imaginations that we never regretted not having a television.

Like the farm, my hobby of collecting World War II memorabilia expanded beyond my expectations. It started with my saving the postcards and insignias that friends in the service used to send to my older sister during the war. Curiosity led me to shows that sell antique toys, books, propaganda posters, and more postcards. My collection has been in a museum show and is featured in a book on the war effort.

Some people ask me how I do it all. It's not that I do *that* much. But the things I have chosen to do happen to satisfy very different parts of myself.

Practicing law provides me with an intellectual challenge, while the farm allows me to be outside, have quiet times, and get great exercise. Collecting is where I satisfy my interest in history and where I can escape to a very different world. This kind of diversity leads to a deep sense of balance and fulfillment. I'm a happy man.

Training His Sights on a Dream

Travis H. P. Prok, Laredo, Texas

Date of birth: May 13, 1967

Profession: Kinesiology instructor and rodeo coach

I believe that there's a special "train" that shows up in everyone's life. If you get on that train, it will take you on a fantastic journey of self-discovery and personal growth. For me, that train has been rodeo. Although I'd always been fascinated by it, I didn't really consider trying it until a special person took the time to encourage me.

We were living in Calgary, Alberta, Canada, at the time, and my mom took it upon herself to call Mount Royal College and speak to the chairman there. He told her that it sounded like her son had a lot of potential. But it wasn't so much having straight A's that would get me somewhere; it was my ability to have the heart to work hard at whatever I pursued. I ended up enrolling in the sports medicine program at Mount Royal College, where the man she spoke with, Dexter Nelson, happened to be the president of the rodeo club. He encouraged me to try a rodeo school. So one day in 1989, I drove about nine hours in this little Chevette to the middle of nowhere to learn bull riding. That three-day weekend turned out to be the most enriching experience I've ever gone through in my entire life. This incredible self-discovery took place, and I realized that I'd found my "train."

As I continued to pursue my schooling in sports medicine, I entered dozens of rodeos, which left me just enough money to live from semester to semester. When I started feeling like I couldn't squeeze another ounce out of a day, I'd just remember how my mom had sacrificed for me. She still is my source of inspiration.

Today, on Monday through Friday, I assume the role of college professor and head rodeo coach at Laredo Community College. When the weekends come, though, I love to hit a rodeo and just unwind and enjoy other facets of my life. My other hat is my entrepreneurial business, Rodeo Kinetics. It serves the rodeo community from a sports-science perspective. I market bull riding equipment and special training apparatuses and do sports-safety, fitness, and motivational seminars. It's my insurance policy to pay the bills and take care of the family that I hope to have some day. I also write a column for *Pro Rodeo World* magazine.

As far as hobbies go, I enjoy any activity that promotes good health and fitness. Right now, I'm taking classes in aikido, which is a Japanese art of self-defense. I also like studying about alternative health remedies and Eastern philosophy. Down the road, I want to try gator hunting—at least just one time.

How do I do it all? There's really no set game plan other than just disciplining myself to make the time for everything, prioritizing stuff, and trying not to be too consumed with any one area. I'm always striving to do better, though, and that's what keeps me motivated. I honestly feel that my life is balanced and fulfilling because I love what I'm doing. But it hasn't been easy. I've always had to work at finding the time, the money, and the discipline. It's a continuous process of growth that requires a lot of patience and effort.

It's all worth it in the end, when you're out there on that bull. You have to find the natural rhythm and timing of that animal and go with it. If you do, it's magical. A dance of perfect harmony with that much power is an incredible experience—like nothing else.

Ultimately, I want to be able to give back to others some of what I've learned. To be able to encourage and mentor someone else who has a low level of self-esteem or had a tough childhood—that's what I want to do. I want to help them find that train and repeat the cycle.

Taking Challenges to New Heights

Lee Vogan,
Cold Lake, Alberta, Canada

Date of birth: April 9, 1963

Profession: F-18 fighter pilot in the Canadian Air Force

I never walk away from a challenge. After graduating from Carleton University in Ottawa with a bachelor's degree in law, I was trying to figure out what to do with my life when my grandfather asked me, "Why don't you join the Air Force?" I just laughed and he replied, "You could be a jet pilot." I thought that sounded kind of cool, but I wasn't the least bit interested in military life. Then he said the magic words: "Maybe they wouldn't take you."

That afternoon I was in the recruiting center signing up.

Now I can't imagine doing anything else. When I strap myself into an F/A 18, it becomes an extension of me. I have the ability to go supersonic, to go vertical, to dive, to roll upside down and stay that way and then do loops and rolls. Besides that, I can fire rockets, drop bombs, or trigger down a cannon that shoots 100 rounds a second. It's a fantastic experience—and a hell of a lot of fun.

Flying a fighter is the kind of job you never master. As soon as I get a handle on one aspect of the job, there's another to be learned. I will retire and still not know all there is to know, especially when it comes to air combat, which is a truly three-dimensional challenge you can never get too good at. Everyday I'm faced with new challenges, and I wouldn't have it any other way.

In this line of work, it certainly helps to be in shape. I work out quite a bit and cycle to work as often as I can. Lifting weights and boxing a heavy bag helps with fitness and reduces stress as well. In general, I try to be pretty active—at my age you really have to.

When I'm not "burning up dinosaurs" and flying "at the speed of heat," my wife and I enjoy taking trips to our cottage in the Rocky Mountains of southern Alberta. While there, we involve ourselves in many outdoor activities such as hiking, skiing, snowmobiling, quading, off-road trucking, swimming, and, of course, fly fishing (the only way to fish!). We also enjoy classic cars and fine wine. I have a couple of cars, but my daily driver is a 1970 GMC half-ton. That's a *man's* vehicle as far as I'm concerned. As for the wine, my wife, Kristy, and I ferment our own.

I tend to live each day like it's my last, which I think is a good philosophy. Life is short and there are so many places, people, and things to see.

Fortunately, my job takes me all over. I've yet to see Newfoundland or Rhode Island but have been pretty much everywhere else in North America. One thing is for sure: Going away for a week each month certainly keeps the magic alive in my marriage. There's no routine, and it's very exciting to see my wife when I return.

We're planning to start a family soon, so fatherhood will be my next challenge. I think when a man is in his midthirties, it's a good time to settle down and start passing on some of the stuff he has learned to somebody else. One thing I want to teach my kids is that when something bad happens to you and it's really upsetting, ask yourself if you're going to look back and laugh about it in 10 years. If the answer is yes (and it usually is), then laugh about it now. Let me tell you, I do a lot of laughing.

I can't express how great it is to be flying high in my job and in life generally. That won't end when I hang up my wings either . . . there's always another challenge around the corner.

Index

Underscored references indicate boxed text. **Boldface** references indicate illustrations or photographs.